GOLDEN KEYS TO
INTERNAL PHYSICAL FITNESS

By Paul C. Bragg, N.D., Ph.D.

LIFE EXTENSION SPECIALIST

with

Patricia Bragg, Ph.D.

HEALTH AND BEAUTY CONSULTANT

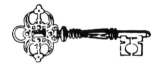

Published by

HEALTH SCIENCE
Box 7, Santa Barbara, California 93102 U.S.A.

GOLDEN KEYS TO INTERNAL PHYSICAL FITNESS

By Paul C. Bragg, N.D., Ph.D.
Life Extension Specialist
and
Patricia Bragg, Ph.D.
Health and Beauty Consultant

Ninth Printing MCMLXXVIII

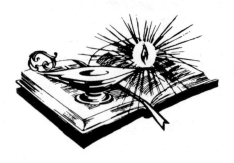

Published in the United States by

HEALTH SCIENCE   Box 7, Santa Barbara, California 93102 U.S.A.

LIBRARY OF CONGRESS
CATALOG CARD NUMBER: 66-30394

ISBN: 0-87790-006-X

PRINTED IN THE UNITED STATES OF AMERICA

ACKNOWLEDGMENTS

As with each of my books and manuscripts, I find myself ever grateful to my daughter Patricia Bragg for her understanding and help in the research, proofreading, typing and evaluation of my writings.

My special gratitude to my loyal and dedicated office staff for their generous assistance.

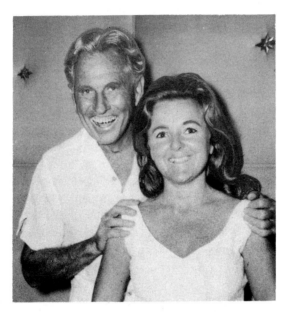

WHY THIS BOOK WAS WRITTEN

Paul and Patricia Bragg have Nutritional Physical Fitness as outlined in this book. They eat Natural Foods as close to Nature as possible. They have a systematic program of exercise, deep breathing, sun-bathing and all the natural hygiene that contributes to building Super Health and Internal Physical Fitness. They believe that man cannot live by bread alone, and that everyone should develop a philosophy of life as outlined in this book.

When you are Healthy you are Happy.

Paul C. Bragg

TOTAL HEALTH FOR THE TOTAL PERSON

In a broad sense, "Total Health for the Total Person" is a combination of physical, mental, emotional, social, and spiritual components. The ability of the individual to function effectively in his environment depends on how smoothly these components function as a whole. Of all the qualities that comprise an integrated personality, a well-developed, totally fit body is one of the most desirable.

A person may be said to be totally physically fit if they function as a total personality with efficiency and without pain or discomfort of any kind. That is to have a Painless, Tireless, Ageless body, possessing sufficient muscular strength and endurance to maintain an effective posture, successfully carries on the duties imposed by the environment, meets emergencies satisfactorily and has enough energy for recreation and social obligations after the "work day" has ended, meets the requirements for his environment through efficient functioning of his sense organs, possesses the resilience to recover rapidly from fatigue, tension, stress and strain without the aid of stimulants, and enjoys natural sleep at night and feels fit and alert in the morning for the job ahead.

Keeping the body totally fit and functional is no job for the uninformed or the careless person. It requires an understanding of the body, sound health and eating practices, and disciplined living. The results of such a regimen can be measured in happiness, radiant health, agelessness, peace of mind, in the joy of living and high achievement.

Paul C. Bragg and Patricia Bragg

"I have found a perfect health, a new state of existence, a feeling of purity and happiness, something unknown to humans . . ."
—Novelist Upton Sinclair,
who fasted frequently.

GOLDEN KEYS TO INTERNAL PHYSICAL FITNESS

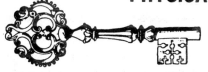

CONTENTS

From the Bragg home to your home we share our years of health knowledge—years of living close to God and Nature and what joys of fruitful, radiant living this produces—this my Father and I share with you and your loved ones.

Patricia Bragg

Contents

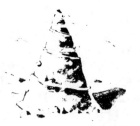

The Endless Quest

Freedom and progress rest in man's continual search for truth.
Truth is the summit of being.

—Emerson

GOLDEN KEYS TO INTERNAL PHYSICAL FITNESS

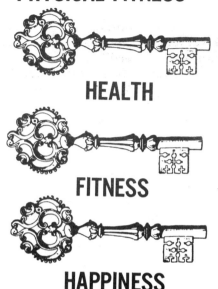

HEALTH

FITNESS

HAPPINESS

HOW TO LIVE LONG ...

STAY HEALTHY ...

AND BE YOUTHFUL

First, and foremost I want you to keep in mind "Vis Medicatrix Naturae," the all-healing power of Nature. The human body is self-repairing and self-healing and self-rejuvenating!

Treat your body correctly and it will be an instrument of joy and happiness, and you will be rewarded with a rich, long life. You will look and feel younger than your years.

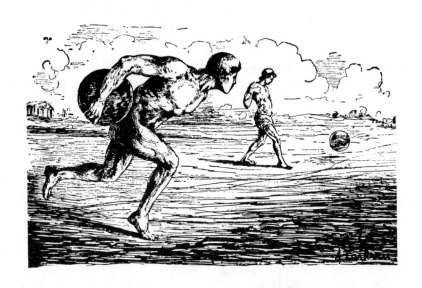

THE WONDER-WORKING WITHIN YOU

Before you read this book I want to talk to *YOU* personally. This is a "heart-to-heart" talk between the reader and the author. First I want *YOU* to bear in mind this one pertinent fact: *YOU CAN ACHIEVE INTERNAL PHYSICAL FIT-NESS.* No matter how hopeless *You* may feel, what poor shape *You* are in, or how old *You* are. I want *You* to definitely know that it is possible for *You* to step out of the present body *You* are now living in and build an entirely new one. *You* can enjoy life again. I emphasize, *YOU CAN DO IT!*

The guidance you need is in this *small book.* The perseverance and courage are within *yourself.* THE STRENGTH TO RECOVER IS WITHIN *YOU*, ONCE YOU ARE SHOWN THE WAY. I assure *YOU* of this.

Each of us has extraordinary *POWER* to accomplish what we demand of ourselves, if we care to search for it. *YOU* are no exception. *YOU* can find it if *YOU* make up your mind to, however great a weakling *YOU* may think yourself at this moment. I have no illusions about *YOU*: I am not writing this book for the rare brave people, but for *YOU*, probably an ordinary being with no more courage than the rest of us. BUT —and this is the important thing—*YOU* have the untapped, unsuspected *POWER* in reserve that the Creator has given to all of us. It is possible that *YOU* may be aware of such power but may feel, because of your poor physical condition, unable to release it. This book will help *YOU* find this *POWER*, and show *YOU* how to release and *USE* it!

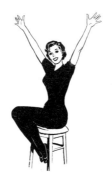

THE PHYSICAL CULTURE CREED

We Believe:

That our body is our most glorious possession; that health-wealth is our greatest asset; that every influence which interferes with the attainment of superb health should be recognized as a menace.

We maintain that weakness is truly a crime; that sickness and premature ageing are the penalties of violated health laws; that every man can be a vigorous specimen of masculinity; that every woman can be a splendidly strong, well-poised specimen of femininity, and look many years younger than her years . . .

IF THE LAWS OF LIFE ARE RIGIDLY OBSERVED.

WE BELIEVE THE REQUIREMENTS IN BUILDING AGELESS HEALTH TO BE:

FIRST: Pure air and sunlight whenever obtainable; thorough ventilation of living rooms.

SECOND: A nutritious and wholesome diet of live vital foods, well masticated, eaten only at the dictates of a normal appetite; frequent fasting of a day or two to give the body a physiological rest ... to give the body a chance to do some house-cleaning. A weekly fast of 24 hours including water only (distilled water preferred) should be part of every true Physical Culture Fitness program.

THIRD: A brisk daily walk of one hour regardless of weather conditions, and practicing full deep breathing as you stride along. Practicing good posture habits with head held high, chest high and stomach drawn in.

FOURTH: Reasonable regular use of the muscular system throughout the entire body in work, home exercises, in the gymnasium, on the athletic field, and elsewhere. No matter what you do in your daily life you need a good, balanced program of exercise which will enable you to become the person you want to be.

FIFTH: Thorough cleanliness, which requires frequent baths—cold baths for a tonic—hot baths for cleanliness. Thorough friction with open hands, brush or towel is also valuable.

SIXTH: Internal cleanliness, which is a matter of regular and thorough elimination.

SEVENTH: Abundant sleep, measured in depth or quality as well as duration; this power of deep sleep being dependent upon sufficient exercise and healthful habits.

EIGHTH: As Physical Culturists we realize that our Universal Life Force is our greatest wealth. We build our Universal Life Force each day by following the natural laws of God and Nature. Universal Life Force cannot be purchased at any price. It must be earned by observing the Natural laws of Health.

NINTH: We believe that we are God's and Nature's perfect children and that our bodies are the Temple of the Living God, therefore we believe that we are Body, Mind and Spirit. We must keep our body well, strong and clean.

TENTH: We believe through Physical Culture we can keep the physical body well and youthful, but that we must build the Inner Strength by depending on a Power higher than ourselves. We believe in prayer and meditation to build Inner Spiritual Strength.

LIFE IS FOR THE LIVING
THE JOY OF LIVING GOES TO THOSE WHO ARE FIT IN BODY, MIND AND SPIRIT

Life is the most precious possession we can have. To enjoy this priceless treasure of living we must have Superior Health —Superior Health that comes from *INTERNAL PHYSICAL FITNESS.*

Most people have completely lost their sense of values. Many think that making big money, buying big cars, owning real estate, stocks, bonds, jewelry, big homes, and acquiring social status and fame are the treasures of life. I will not discount any of these attainments, but they are worth very little when you are sick, half-sick, run-down and physically out of shape. How can you enjoy *anything* when you feel wretched in every cell of your body?

What good is his material wealth when a man is told that his life will be finished at 66.6 years? (which is the life expectancy of the average American male.) And how can an American female enjoy her possessions when her life is expected to be over at 73.4 years?

11

Certainly our skidding national fitness statistics and the mounting incidence of premature obituaries indicate cause for general alarm. But so far neither the federal government nor any other organization has done a great deal towards getting the premature ageing, soft, flabby, out of shape, indolent American off his backside.

THE YOUNG ARE DOOMED

It was Bernard Shaw who said, "Youth is wasted on the young." This is certainly a true statement. Except for a few intelligent young people, it is practically impossible to get the American youth interested in Internal Physical Fitness. You may challenge this by saying, "Look at all the young men and women engaged in athletic sports, in tennis, surf-boarding and all the other activities." But as a man with long experience in physical culture in all its branches, I must explain to you that athletics and sports are not the answer to Internal Physical Fitness. It requires much more than athletics and sports to build solid physical fitness. It is not only exercise but also good nutrition, rest, relaxation and Mind-Power that build Internal Physical Fitness.

The young never think of tomorrow or next year or ten or twenty years from now. The young want to dynamite the treasure vaults of life. "Live it up today; tomorrow may never come!" is the motto of the young. "Eat, drink and be merry" —and away they go, burning themselves out with tobacco, alcohol, L.S.D. and other poisons for kicks, late hours, sluggishness and, of course, plenty of meaningless sex. But tomorrow *does* come, and what shape does it find them in?

Yes, youth is wasted on the young. They smash through the red danger lights of life but when they reach middle-age (middle-age is between 40 and 60), they are forced to slow down, all arrogance gone, and their banner which read "BORN TO RAISE HELL" is rotted and turned to ashes.

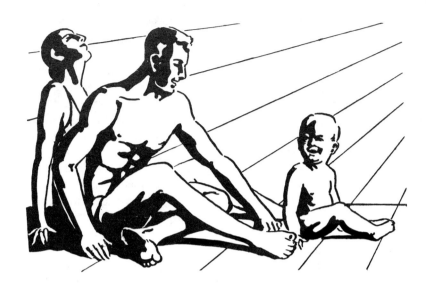

HOW GOOD ARE WE WHEN IT
COMES TO LONG LIFE?

So, the wild youth of twenty years ago is the middle-aged of today. Do you know that by the time a person reaches 40 he has lived over half his life? Don't forget the life expectancy of man is 66.6 years and a female 73.4 years in the United States.

Oh, we are constantly told what great health we have, and how we have added years to our lives. Yes, our new-born babies survive longer because of good common-sense and cleanliness. They have made the figures look very interesting.

A baby born in 1975 can be expected to live 23 years longer than one born in 1900. Yet a young man today, just out of college or the service and presumably in the best physical condition, has only eight years greater life expectancy than his grandfather had at the same age.

Today's unfit American is in infinitely worse shape to avoid or survive infectious diseases, heart attacks or strokes than were his grandparents. His grandparents ate a more natural diet and were more active physically. We have many diseases of degeneration that his grandfather never heard about. He was a much more relaxed person. He was not tormented by stresses, strains and tension as our men are today. He led a more carefree life getting pleasure and joy out of the simple things of life. He moved at a much slower pace . . . took time to look up at the stars at night . . . to enjoy the glories of a sunrise and the beauties of a sunset. He enjoyed long hikes in the out-of-doors. He went to bed earlier and met the dawn with gladness in his heart and an appreciation of the good life.

The lack of sanitation was his greatest enemy. This is what killed him. He didn't know how to keep his drinking water clean and free of pollution. He did not have the wonders of refrigeration, thus he often ate spoiled food. Sanitation and cleanliness have contributed very greatly to adding these eight years.

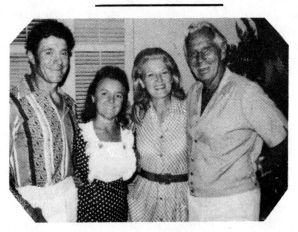

Jack LaLanne, Patricia Bragg, Elaine LaLanne & Paul Bragg

Jack says, "Bragg saved my life at age 14 when I attended the Bragg Health & Fitness Lecture in Oakland, California." From that day on, Jack has lived the health life and teaches Health & Fitness to millions every morning with his T.V. Exercise Show.

A RANK LIST OF LIFE EXPECTANCY

The following table lists countries with the world's longest life expectancies. In the column at left, which gives the average life expectancy of men (from birth), the United States ranks 18th. At right are the figures for women (the United States ranks 10th).

LIFE EXPECTANCY IN YEARS

MEN			WOMEN
Netherlands	71.4	75.4	Sweden
Sweden	71.3	75.0	Iceland
Norway	71.1	74.8	Netherlands
Israel	70.9	74.8	Switzerland
Iceland	70.7	74.7	Norway
Denmark	70.4	74.2	Canada
Switzerland	69.5	74.1	France
Canada	68.4	73.9	England & Wales
New Zealand	68.2	73.8	Denmark
England & Wales	68.0	73.4	United States
Spain	67.3	73.0	U.S.S.R.
Puerto Rico	67.3	73.0	Israel
Czechoslovakia	67.2	73.0	New Zealand
France	67.2	72.8	Czechoslovakia
Japan	67.2	72.8	Australia
Australia	67.1	72.4	West Germany
West Germany	66.9	72.3	Japan
United States	66.6	72.1	Puerto Rico

OUR LIVES ARE SO SHORT

15

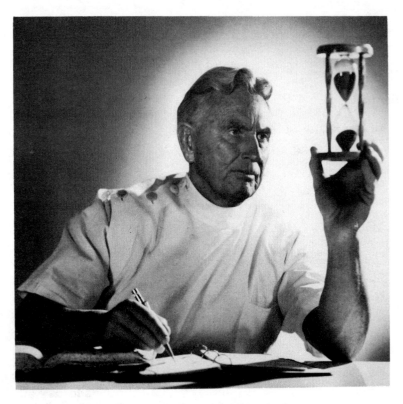

Paul Bragg asks "How long will you live?"

"Men do not die, they KILL themselves."
—Seneca, Roman Philosopher

Whatsoever was the father of a disease; an ill diet was the mother.
— Herbert, 1859

Many people go throughout life committing partial suicide — destroying their health, youth, beauty, talents, energies, creative qualities. Indeed, to learn how to be good to oneself is often more difficult than to learn how to be good to others.

If a man can convince me that I do not think or act right, gladly will I change, for I search after truth. But he is harmed who abideth on still in his ignorance.
— Marcus Aurelius, Roman Emperor

OUR LIVES ARE SO SHORT

Figures do not lie. They are hard and cold. But they give a truthful picture, vividly pointing out that we stand before the world with the lowest life expectancy of 18 of the countries of the world.

Just think of it! A man today has only 66.6 years to live and a woman only 73.4 years. Do you believe that this is the normal span of human life?

To me, a man who has lived to my present age, these are *tragic* figures! I have lived many years over the average life expectancy and I expect to reach 120 years or more in a superior state of radiant health. I know that nothing can kill me except disease...and I know that if I follow the natural health laws of life, I am not going to get a disease. How is it possible for a man like myself to contract a disease when I keep myself in the very best *INTERNAL PHYSICAL FITNESS?*

There are no diseases that strike just because a person has reached a certain age. Diseases must have causes! But senility and premature ageing are caused by not knowing the laws of Nature! We are punished by our bad habits of living and rewarded by our good habits. This is what the golden keys to internal physical fitness will give you ... a plan of healthful living so you can laugh as you joyously watch the birthdays slip by.

Correct diet can lay the foundation for a longer life span ... systematic exercise can help make this foundation a durable structure!

A BREAK-DOWN OF THE KILLERS
WHICH ATTACK THE UNFIT

Life is the survival of the fittest. To attain long life without landing in a hospital, a convalescent rest home or a mental institution we must fight for our health and life.

We can never drop our guard. Self-preservation is the first law of life. We have many vicious enemies that are waiting to destroy us. Woe to the weak—for they will perish long before their time.

Here I present the sad figures of our enemies. These are the killers who are just waiting for us to let our bodies weaken so they can pounce on us and make us suffer and then butcher us in cold blood.

THE MAJOR CAUSES OF DEATH

Latest figures on the 15 leading Causes of Death (excluding prenatal deaths).

Causes of Death	Number of Deaths	% Total Deaths
Coronary Heart Disease	707,830	39.0
Cancer	291,870	15.7
Stroke	201,166	11.1
Accidents (Auto and Other)	100,669	5.6
Influenza and Pneumonia	70,761	3.9
Diseases of Early Infancy	62,688	3.5
General Arteriosclerosis (Hardening of the Arteries)	37,429	2.1
Diabetes	32,465	1.8
Circulatory Diseases	24,385	1.3
Lung Diseases	23,205	1.3
Cirrhosis of the Liver	22,456	1.2
Suicide	20,840	1.1
Congenital Malformations	20,817	1.1
Hypertensive Diseases	12,694	0.7
Ulcer of Stomach and Duodenum	12,161	0.7
All other Causes	172,112	9.9

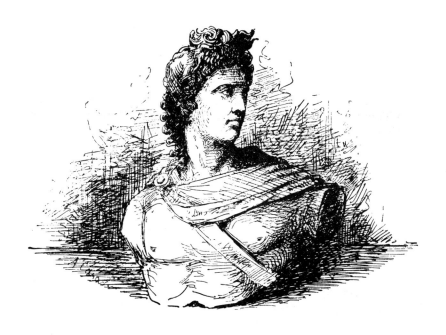

THE RISE AND FALL OF A HUMAN

Seventy-five years still falls far short of what we may reasonably consider to be the human span of life. But many are doomed to fall by the wayside long before their journey through life has been completed. Just how many will fall in this way, how many "last the course," and how long that course is, can be best understood by looking at the Life Tables. Superficially these tables may appear to be rather dull masses of figures, of interest only to statisticians. Actually they are fascinating, for behind them lies the whole drama of human life, of birth, growth, maturation, ageing, accident, disease, and death in all its forms. They portray the rise and fall of the great arc of life and, though they cannot answer our question regarding the real length of the human life span, they can at least give us some indications.

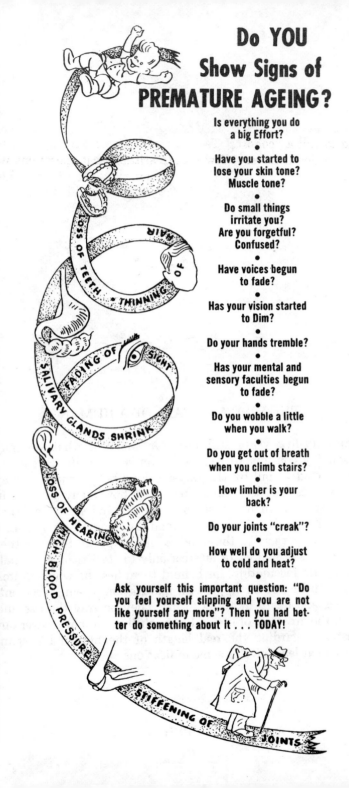

Do YOU Show Signs of PREMATURE AGEING?

Is everything you do
a big Effort?

•

Have you started to
lose your skin tone?
Muscle tone?

•

Do small things
irritate you?
Are you forgetful?
Confused?

•

Have voices begun
to fade?

•

Has your vision started
to Dim?

•

Do your hands tremble?

•

Has your mental and
sensory faculties begun
to fade?

•

Do you wobble a little
when you walk?

•

Do you get out of breath
when you climb stairs?

•

How limber is your
back?

•

Do your joints "creak"?

•

How well do you adjust
to cold and heat?

Ask yourself this important question: "Do
you feel yourself slipping and you are not
like yourself any more"? Then you had better do something about it . . . TODAY!

In Table 1 is shown an abbreviated form of the Life Tables taken from the figures published by the National Office of Vital Statistics. The table assumes that we have started with 100,000 newborn babies. This is quite a lot of babies, and represents a large sample of the population which statisticians like to call a "cohort." To these 100,000 we have applied the known death rates. A few simple arithmetical operations will enable us to forecast (1) how many members of our cohort will die in a given year, (2) for how many years the remainder can, on the average, expect to survive.

To make the example more concrete we will assume that we are able at intervals to assemble our "cohort" and to note its progress along the road of life.

LIFE TABLE
100,000 newborn babies

Age of Cohort	Number of Deaths	Number of Survivors	Life Expectancy of Survivors
1	2,722	97,278	69.02
10	766	96,502	61.48
20	739	95,763	51.91
30	1,227	94,536	42.52
40	1,920	92,616	33.29
50	4,506	88,110	24.70
60	10,004	78,006	17.15
70	18,887	59,189	10.89
80	28,751	30,438	6.27
90	24,237	6,201	3.41
100	6,005	196	1.92
105	184	12	1.53
110	11	1	—

Every man is the builder of a temple called his body . . . We are all sculptors and painters, and our material is our own flesh, blood and bones. Any nobleness begins at once to refine a man's features, any meanness or sensuality to imbrute them.
— Henry David Thoreau

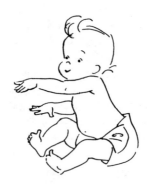

THE JOURNEY OF LIFE BEGINS

To begin with, here are our 100,000 newborns, males and females, all born, let us say, on June 1, 1950. These 100,000 newborns are not new lives, for it is merely a convention, and, biologically speaking, a very unsound convention, that accepts birth as the starting point of life. Actually, of course, life started for our cohort some nine months earlier, when a single sperm penetrated an egg, fused with its nucleus, and set the life in motion.

Biologically speaking, those first nine months were the most vitally important period in the life of our cohort, a period of almost unbelievable activity in the course of which one microscopic egg cell multiplied to form a baby of about 26 million million cells. Surprisingly enough the growing embryo, long before it was ready to emerge from the womb, had already undergone certain losses, had, in fact, aged in the sense that ageing is loss. The chief of these losses was the gill clefts of which every human embryo develops a set memory of the old days when all life was confined to the waters, and gills were the established means of breathing. Naturally it is desirable that the embryo should lose its gill clefts since the infant might otherwise be uncertain as to whether it was a man or a fish. But this very early degeneration and loss of an organ suggests that the ageing process begins, in a sense, before we are even born.

We must realize also that our 100,000 newborns are survivors of a greater population of fertilized eggs, many of which never got so far as birth. Many an embryo is lost during the first few months of pregnancy, many a fetus is aborted during the later months (about 16.2 per 1000 according to a recent estimate). Our cohort, however, has at least contrived to survive long enough to get itself a birth certificate. We will now follow its destiny from this point.

FIRST BIRTHDAY PARTY

We will assemble our cohort for the first time when it has completed one year of life outside the womb. Diaper days are still with the little creatures and they display the chubby contours of the very young. They are rich in moisture, not as rich as they were when in the womb, but still very moist. This accounts for their plumpness and for the smoothness of their skin. Through their rosy gums the first crop of teeth is just beginning to burst. They weigh on the average twenty-three pounds and are twenty-nine inches tall.

So there they are, the hundred thousand, laughing, gurgling, toddling, bawling, doing all those things that one-year-olds delight in. One hundred thousand? No. We have forgotten to count them, and when we do so we may be shocked at the total. Death has already been busy and reaped a sizable crop. Even in these days of highly developed infant care and in this very hygienic United States of America, 2,722 of our babies have perished. Two thousand seven hundred and twenty-two small coffins ... The death rate in the first year of life is scandalously high. So actually there are 97,278 babies at our first birthday party. On the average they can expect to live a further 69.02 years, 67.41 if they are males, 72.77 if they are females.

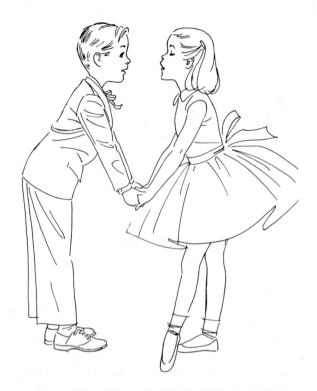

HAPPY BIRTHDAY, TEN-YEAR OLDS!

When our cohort next celebrates together it is 1960. We no longer have gurgling, toddling, bawling diaper-wetters but frisky ten-year-olds, school children, full of games and tricks. Their "baby teeth" are all gone. The set they now have must last for the rest of their lives. They have grown in height and weight, the boys are 54.5 inches tall and weigh on the average 70.4 pounds, the girls are 54.4 and weigh 70.2 pounds. And their numbers? There are 96,502 of them. The reaper has been relatively idle and felled only 776 in the nine years which have elapsed since our last birthday party. The survivors can look forward on the average to 61.48 years more life.

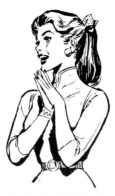

TODAY YOU ARE TWENTY!

Again a decade elapses. 1970. Once more our cohort assembles. What a change this time! Childhood is over; the beings who have gathered for this twentieth birthday party are young men and women, not legally of age it is true, but independent and beyond parental control. During the past ten years one of the great biological road markers has been passed. The message has gone out from the mysterious timekeeper that resides, apparently, in the pituitary gland. Roused by gonadotropic hormones, the sex glands, ovaries in the females, testes in the males, have started to pour their sex hormones into the blood stream. So the girls are not only menstruating and ovulating but carry the other badges of developed womanhood, the rounded breasts, and characteristic hair on the pubis, the softer smoother contours of the female. The males, stimulated by testosterone rather than estradiol, have witnessed a growth of their sexual apparatus from infantile to mature dimensions. They have experienced the sudden upsurge of desire which is the inevitable accompaniment of these changes.

It is in this decade from ten to twenty years that the death rate sinks to a minimum. Only 739 members of our cohort have perished, most of them as a result of accidents which take a high toll of the males in this age group. The 95,763 survivors can expect, on the average, 51.91 years more life. Even at this relatively early age the greater power to survive of the female reflects itself in the predominance of females.

THAT THIRTIETH BIRTHDAY:
TIME TO THINK

On June 1, 1980 we once again assemble our cohort. We now have men and women of thirty, most of them married and already parents. They are young by our present-day standards but already the time of greatest vigor and of maximum sexual activity is over, at least for the male. The change is too slight to be noticed except in those who make a living by particularly strenuous forms of activity. The professional baseball player or boxer will know by the time his thirtieth birthday arrives that the ageing process has been at work, that his reactions are just a little slower than they were. Other members of our cohort will still consider themselves in the prime of life, as indeed they are. The decade they have left behind has seen relatively few deaths; 1,227 to be exact. It leaves us with 94,536 survivors each having an expectation of 42.52 more years of life.

DOES LIFE BEGIN AT FORTY?

When we next gather our cohort, in the year 1990, its members have reached a turning point. The fortieth year marks the beginning of the decline; the great arc of life has passed its zenith and from now on must travel a descending curve. They have arrived at middle-age . . . 40 to 60.

Those destined to get rich are wealthy already, those doomed to success have probably had their first taste of that potent intoxicant, those destined to fail have already gone far in failure.

Yet there will be some in our cohort who have not, even at forty, reached the height of their powers.

This applies particularly to those who have lived on a natural diet, have taken vigorous daily exercises and have kept themselves Internally Physically Fit. Instead of cracking-up they are enjoying agelessness. They are in perfect physical shape. They look younger than their years. They feel just as strong and vigorous as they did at 25. They are entering middle-age alive and alert with a tireless, painless and ageless body. But the average cohort now suffers from chronic fatigue and many other tormenting ailments. To blunt the pain of an unfit body, they nip at a whisky bottle or take different drugs to dull their pains.

(Alcoholism climbs a steep 50% in the 40-60 group over ages 30-39). Their medicine cabinet begins to look like a pharmaceutical display, and they retreat into hypochondria. Indeed, their bad living habits contribute to the cardiovascular and cardiopulmonary attacks that increasingly kill the middle-agers.

The middle-ager is full of aches and pains. The dietetic deficiencies and the sins of laziness start to show around forty and they will increase as the years go by. Half of their life is over and as they look down the corridor of life it looks dark and gloomy. They laughed at the person who was health-minded—called him a "Health crank" and a "Health faddist." But the laughs are all gone now as they are too busy telling others about their aches and pains. The next 20 years (if they live) are going to be sad and painful.

As for their physical appearance, many of our forty-year olds are already carrying a little too much weight, and physical deterioration has probably progressed futher than it need have done. Many are already gray and many of the faces are heavily lined. The women in particular know that their battle with the encroaching wrinkles cannot much longer be fought with any hope of victory. The ovaries, almost exhausted, produce eggs which seem to have lost much of their innate vigor, and reproduction, once the fortieth year has been reached, becomes more perilous both for mother and child. Death has harvested a larger crop in this fourth decade, 1,920 members of our cohort have died which leaves us with 92,616 survivors each having life expectancy of 33.29 more years.

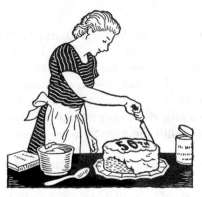

CELEBRATE THE HALF-CENTURY

Our birthday party for fifty-year-olds in the year 2000 shows those changes which were already apparent ten years earlier in a somewhat more obvious form. The wrinkles are more pronounced, the heads are a little grayer, a little balder, the abdomens tend to be a little more protuberant. The females have definitely given up trying to look like their own daughters and many have passed once and for all out of the reproductive phase of their existence, ceasing either to menstruate or to ovulate. Death has harvested a larger crop, carrying off 4,506, more than twice as many as it did in the previous decade. This leaves 88,110 members of our cohort still alive and gives them, on the average, an expectation of 24.7 more years of life.

SIXTY—AND STAGGERING RESPONSIBILITIES

At our seventh gathering in 2010 we see little change, for the rate of ageing slows as time passes and toward the end of life its progress is very slow. So our sixty-year-olds differ little in appearance from our fifty-year-olds. We can safely assume that all the women are now out of the reproductive phase of life and a large number of them are now grandmothers. As for the men, they have lost much of their libido though several well-preserved specimens may still be capable of fairly vigorous sexual function. Mental power is on the decline. Memory for recent events may be impaired. But wide experience compensates for these losses and many of our sixty-year-olds carry staggering responsibilities. Death has been busier than ever before and has harvested a total of 10,004. The major killers, cardiovascular disease and cancer, are becoming more and more prevalent. Our cohort, however, still contains 78,006 people and each can expect 17.15 more years of life.

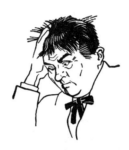

SEVENTY—A PSYCHOLOGICAL VACUUM

Once again we assemble. It is now 2020 and the cohort has reached its seventieth year. Behind lies a critical decade for many of the men. During its first half they carried the maximum load of responsibility, for it is to these men in their early sixties that society most often offers positions of the greatest importance. Then, at sixty-five, many of these responsible executives, administrators, professors, find themselves abruptly shorn alike of their burdens and of their incentives, cast into a psychological vacuum in which they must molder till death brings them release. Death, of course, has been very busy during this decade and harvested a crop of 18,877, leaving 59,189 with an average expectation of 10.89 more years of life.

EIGHTY CANDLES ON THE CAKE

At our next gathering in 2030 we can witness many of the more extreme effects of ageing. About 40 per cent of our eighty-year-olds are invalids, disabled by arthritis, heart disease, hypertension, paralysis agitans, and "strokes" of varying degrees of severity. Many are partially or totally blind and deaf. A large number are mentally unsound. Even so there are still plenty of lively well-preserved people in our cohort who can say as did Adam in *As You Like It*, "Therefore my age is as a lusty winter, frosty but kindly." As for numbers, we have now seen our cohort pass through the decade in which death's harvest reaches a maximum; 28,751 have perished, 30,438 remain with an expectancy on the average of 6.27 more years.

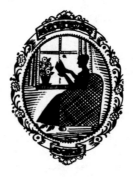

NOW YOU ARE NINETY!

From this point, the decline of our cohort is swift. The group of ancients that assembles on their ninetieth birthday in 2040 certainly shows the effects of ageing to almost the fullest possible extent. Some are still hale and hearty, well-preserved both in body and mind; but many are shrunken, bent, blind, arthritic and peevish, useless to themselves, a burden to their relatives. Their number has fallen dramatically. Death's harvest in this decade was 24,237: 6,201 have survived and can expect on the average 3.41 more years.

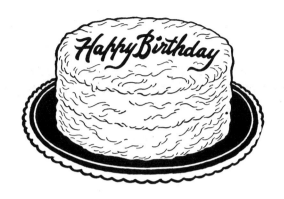

HAPPY BIRTHDAY, CENTENARIAN
WHOEVER YOU ARE

At our next gathering only 196 of our original 100,000 remain alive. It is now 2050, just one hundred years since the day they were born. At this stage in our cohort's progress through time, the superior survival power of the female over the male becomes particularly evident. Of our 196 centenarians 140 are women and only 56 are men. They can expect, on the average, 1.92 years more life.

ONE LONELY SURVIVOR TO BLOW
THE CANDLES OUT

The story is almost ended. In 2055 we find twelve of our original cohort still living at the age of one hundred and five. By 2060 eleven of these have perished. One lonely survivor has reached the age of one hundred and ten.

LIVE THE NATURAL HEALTH LIFE TO SURVIVE

So the drama is ended. The last grave has been dug, the last coffin has been lowered into it. It is the year 2061 and of our original cohort not one remains. What have we learned from the pattern of their lives and the distribution of their deaths?

These cohorts did not die, they killed themselves because they did not know the science of INTERNAL PHYSICAL FITNESS. If these 100,000 persons could have lived by the principles of the book you now hold in your hand, the whole story would have to be rewritten. Many of them would have lived to 100. Many would have reached 120 and longer—and while they lived they would have enjoyed a superior state of living. They would have had strong eyes all the days of their lives. Instead of being stiff and crippled-up with pain they would have had a supple and youthful body for a 100 years or more.

WHAT ABOUT YOUR LIFE?

The book you hold in your hand will give you the Golden Keys to Internal Physical Fitness—from this second on, *YOU* with *MIND-POWER* are going to make a wonderful life for yourself. Read this book—reread it—study it. It is going to give you the knowledge and wisdom to begin an exciting new youthful life.

UNCOMPLICATE YOUR LIVING

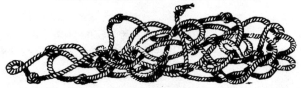

Living is a continual lesson in problem solving, but the trick is to know where to start. No excuses — start your Health Program Today.

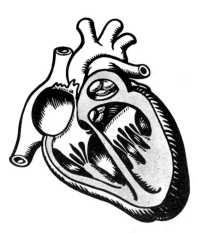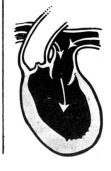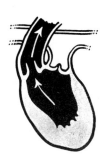

THE HEART AND ITS VALVES

The upper diagram shows the heart cut across to reveal the
Ventricles with their valves. The lower diagram illustrates
the action of the Valves of the Left Ventricle.

YOU WILL LEARN HOW DEADLY "RUST" FROM WRONG EATING AND LACK OF EXERCISE CAN STOP YOUR HEART LONG BEFORE YOUR TIME

From this book you are going to learn how to take care of
your heart. The human heart is perhaps the world's most
fantastic machine. It is about the size of a fist and weighs
less than one pound. It pumps every day the equivalent of
5,500 quarts of blood, weighing about six tons, over more than
60,000 miles of the human circulatory system.

In an average lifetime, the heart beats two and a half
billion times (resting only between beats) and moves 75
million gallons of blood with its life-sustaining oxygen and
nutrients.

To nourish its own muscular tissue during this terrific
effort, the heart itself requires a large quantity of blood,
which flows through the two coronary arteries and their
branches which encircle the heart in a vital network. This
book is going to teach you how to have a healthy heart that
will beat perfectly for 120 years or more.

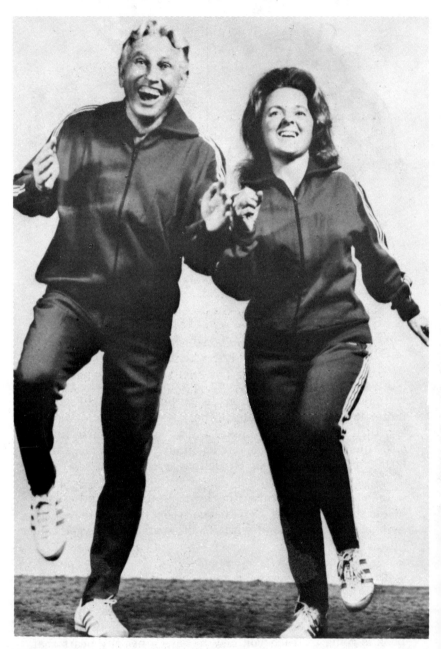

Paul Bragg and daughter Patricia look forward to their daily jogging sessions wherever they are — even with jetting around the world on their health crusades — they enjoy stationary jogging on the big DC-10's and the "747" huge jets, plus it gives them ample room for walking, stretching and keeping limber. Most people arrive at their destination stiff from too much sitting. Don't let this happen to you — enjoy exercising no matter where you may be.

HOW TO BUILD AND MAINTAIN
A POWERFUL HEART

In a healthy heart, the lining of the coronary arteries is clean and smooth. In an unhealthy heart, the arterial walls are thickened and rough. This thickening is caused predominantly by the slow deposit of a fatty wax called cholesterol, which, like rust in a pipe, reduces the flow of blood to the heart tissues.

The reduced flow becomes a serious problem when wrong diet, lack of vigorous exercise or a number of other factors, shown on the following pages, also raise the oxygen demands of the heart. A sudden call for more oxygen—unmet because the blood cannot get through narrowed arteries—can cause a heart attack—a number one killer as you see in the chart.

This book is to help you have a strong and powerful clean heart. *The Golden Keys to Internal Physical Fitness* is your blueprint to a heart that will keep you active for years and years to come. Don't let others criticize you in your fight for a healthy survival. They are not qualified to tell you how to keep Internally Physically Fit. Tell them to live their own life and let you live yours. You may have to do it alone. But be assured if you live by the teachings of this book, you will bury everyone you know who lives a haphazard life. Nature knows no mercy. You must obey her laws or you perish. Nature has no favorites. All are treated alike: the rich and the poor. It is impossible to circumvent the laws of Nature. Obey or die.

Start now. Use the GOLDEN KEYS TO INTERNAL PHYSICAL FITNESS to live 120 years in Health and Happiness.

● You can do it.

    ● Prolong your youth!

        ● Defeat premature ageing!

WHEN YOU ARE HEALTHY — YOU ARE HAPPY!

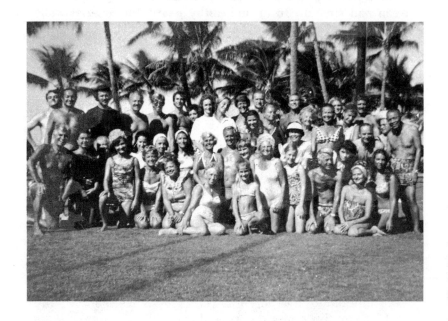

JOIN THE FUN AT THE "LONGER LIFE, HEALTH AND HAPPINESS CLUB" WHEN YOU VISIT HAWAII

Paul and Patricia Bragg and some of their prize members of the "Longer Life, Health and Happiness Club" at their exercise compound at Fort DeRussy, right at Waikiki Beach, Honolulu, Hawaii. Membership is free and open to everyone who wishes to attend any morning Monday through Saturday from 8:30 a.m. to 10:30 a.m. for deep breathing, exercising, meditation, group singing and mini health lectures on how to live a long, healthy life! The group averages 75 to 100 per day. When they are away lecturing they have their leaders carry on until their return. Thousands have visited the club from around the world and then they carry the message of health and happiness to their friends and relatives back home. Paul and Patricia extend an invitation to you and your friends to join the club for health and happiness fellowship with them . . . when you visit Hawaii!

INTERNAL FITNESS GOES DEEPER THAN
APPEARANCE

It is a characteristic of the people in this country to approach the problem of physical fitness from the outside in, and never to go farther in than skin-deep. The average person would be happy to be free from aches and pains, to have a slim, trim waistline and a good coat of tan, and to let it go at that.

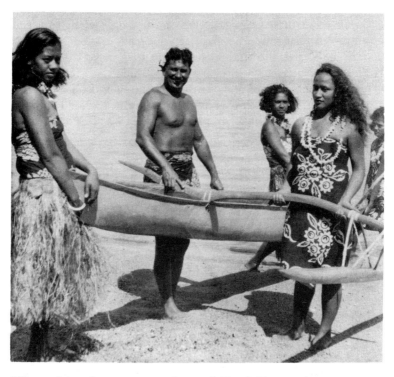

When this picture was taken of Paul Bragg (center) with natives of Tahiti, where he was conducting early research on Physical Fitness, that South Sea Island was a remote, little known spot. Bragg's studies, lectures and writings over the period of some 65 years have taken him to the far corners of the world. . . and have helped many thousands to find the Golden Keys to Physical Fitness.

No one will deny that a good figure and an attractive youthful complexion are desirable. But they are important, not because they contribute to an attractive youthful appearance, but because they reflect an internal well-being that is far more important.

A person who allows his physical condition to deteriorate robs himself of more than an attractive, youthful appearance. He actually endangers his health and his life.

So, in this course of instructions we not only want to teach you how to recapture the glow of youth again—but we want you to have the internal fitness that makes you enjoy the Higher Health. Health in every drop of blood in your body— health and the feeling of youthfulness in every cell and vital organ of your body. You can recapture this higher health if you will allow the natural recuperative forces of the body sufficient play.

Bear that in mind, that your natural recuperative forces can rebuild you back to radiant Health and the feeling of Youthfulness—regardless of your age.

Your body will work for you if you will give it the proper food, if you will exercise it so that you have a strong, sound circulatory system, and if you will learn how to rest and relax it, and not let your emotions and worries drag you down! I promise you it will be a priceless instrument of health and long life. Please, have confidence and faith in the healing power of Nature.

FIRST: STOP POISONING YOUR BODY

You cannot have internal fitness if you persist in putting into your body the dead, devitalized foods and drinks. You should not make a *GARBAGE DISPOSAL OF YOUR STOMACH.*

This very minute let me ask you this personal question. How much slop and dead food did you put in your wonderful body today? How much coffee? Remember there is absolutely NO nourishment in coffee. No nutrients—no vitamins—no minerals—nothing but poisons: deadly caffeine, tars and deadly toxic acids. Tea—how much did you drink today? It has four deadly poisons, and like coffee, no nutrients of any kind. Alcohol? How much of this deadly drink did you put into your body? Cola and soft drinks? How much of this slop did you burden your body with today? How much deadly salt ... and food loaded with this death dealer? How much dead food did you insult your body with ɔday? How much weak, flabby white bread and white sugar 'id you consume? You can't make a garbage disposal of your stomach and·yet expect to have Internal Physical Fitness.You are what you eat. You cannot build super health on trash foods and drinks.

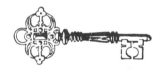

THE GOLDEN KEY—NATURAL DIET

Eat more natural foods, more combination salads with a wide variety of such raw vegetables as cabbage, carrots, celery, grated beets, tomatoes, radishes, parsley, avocado, and watercress. Raw vegetables are a "must" if you expect to have Internal Physical Fitness and raw fruits, too. These are God's and Nature's real foods, filled with the nourishing and purifying natural food chemicals. Properly cooked vegetables (baked vegetables are the best) are essential. You should eat a green cooked vegetable and a yellow cooked vegetable every day of your life. Your blood and body cells need properly cooked vegetables.

And for your protein, you can choose from lean meat, fish, poultry, eggs, natural cheese, raw nuts and nut butters, brewer's yeast, raw wheat germ, soya beans, and dried cooked beans. You have a very wide selection of both animal and vegetarian protein. Plan your meals so that every few weeks you will have at least one serving of each of these proteins.

And your bread—always choose 100% whole grain breads —and that goes for cereals, too. Keep away from Supermarket dry and prepared cereals because they have been "murdered." You should only use 100% freshly ground whole grains for your cereals, and immediately refrigerate them. Rye bread, corn bread, natural brown rice, millet and wholewheat are the foods that are rich in the B Complex vitamins. Make it a hard, fast principle of your life to live on foods as close to nature as possible. Be careful of packaged and prepared foods. Man has put his filthy hands on them and extracted the natural goodness. Read labels . . . if the product is not a 100% natural food, *DON'T EAT IT!*

Building a natural diet is a simple procedure . . . don't try to complicate it. Eat your food as close to nature and the original state as possible, and with the least amount of preparation. Keep your meals simple. Avoid complicated cooking. Replace those over-rich desserts with dates, sun-dried apricots, figs, prunes, and raisins. Your desserts should consist of the natural sweets of life. This is good nutrition in a nut shell. If you eat plenty of raw salads and fruit, you will be supplying the precious minerals and vitamins plus many other nutrients your body needs. Remember, simplicity - natural foods - no unnecessary peeling - no over-cooking.

REVERSE THE PREMATURE AGEING PROCESS
BY VIGOROUS EXERCISE

First, don't tell me you are too old to exercise ... the older you get, the more exercise you need to keep the circulation system of your body in good working order. The more you exercise, the more efficient is your breathing, your heart action, your muscular and joint flexibility, your circulation, your strength and your stamina and endurance.

When you stop exercising and cease to be an active person physically, you soon start slipping physically! You are headed for the human trash heap. I have learned that it is possible for almost anyone, at any age, to undo damage that may have been done through the neglect of exercising and being active physically. It is possible to regain the sort of physical condition that makes life fully worth living. Furthermore, not only is it in your power to earn "more life for your years," it is possible to gain "more long years for your life." I believe every person should live 100 years or more, in contrast to the 66.6 years that is now estimated from actual data.

What I have done for thousands of my health-students over the world, anyone can do for himself, at home, by strictly following this course of instructions to the letter. The first thing you have to do is face the fact that there are no shortcuts to Internal Physical Fitness. There are no crash diets, no special juice drinks, no treatments to give it to you. There are no "dynamic fantastic plans" which will build you up in a short time.

It will take at least four months of hard work ... perhaps the hardest of your entire life, before you see any significant change. So, before you start on this program, you must really WANT to improve your physical fitness. Put everything you have in this course of instructions. You will be proud of yourself and the benefits you will receive.

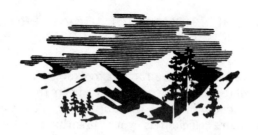

TEN HEALTH COMMANDMENTS

Thou shall respect thy body as the highest manifestation of Life.

Thou shall abstain from all unnatural, devitalized food and stimulating beverages.

Thou shall nourish thy body with only Natural, unprocessed, "live" food, —that

Thou shall extend thy years in health for loving, charitable service.

Thou shall regenerate thy body by the right balance of activity and rest.

Thou shall purify thy cells, tissue and blood with pure fresh air and sunshine.

Thou shall abstain from ALL food when out of sorts in mind or body.

Thou shall keep thy thoughts, words and emotions, pure, calm and uplifting.

Thou shall increase thy knowledge of Nature's laws, abide therewith, and enjoy the fruits of thy life's labor.

Thou shall lift up thyself and thy brother with thine own obedience to ALL Nature's laws.

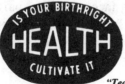

"Teach me Thy way, O Lord;
and lead me in a plain path . . ."
Psalms 97:11

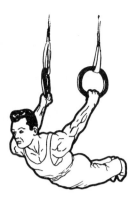

VIGOROUS EXERCISE BUILDS NEW YOUTHFUL BODIES

One of the most spectacular ways of rejuvenating the appearance of the body is by the correct use of the muscles. *The muscles are all ready for use!* They can be put to work without elaborate preparations, merely by the influence of the mind, and when properly organized, they can perform seeming miracles. They can reshape the body, they can lift sagging cheeks, melt away double chins, middle-aged spread, "spare tires," and abdominal bulges. They restore elasticity to the skin, and make it smooth and healthy. They "iron out" crepey necks. They dispose of flabbiness. Flabbiness is a sign of weak, wasted muscles; and wasted muscle can cause premature old age.

The right use of the muscles is one of the great secrets of Internal Physical Fitness, feeling youthful and enjoying superior health. The muscles have an enormously important job: they are the principle weight-carriers of the body; they support the vital organs. Poor or failing eyesight can be due to slackening of the muscles of the face and eyes, particularly, those surrounding the eyes. The "set" of the eye in its socket can be affected by muscular deterioration. Strain results as the eye struggles to accommodate itself.

When we are young, if we are in normal health, we have a natural urge to use our muscles. We want to play games, skip, run, hop, dance, walk, and so on. As we get older, into the thirties the pace slows up. Not only are we (most of us that is) less energetic, but we use our muscles less energetically for those movements we make. When we walk, we tend to make just enough effort to get along; we do not, generally speaking, use our legs from hip to toe as they were made to be used so that all the muscles are brought into play. As a result, the muscles weaken ... then fat forms - flabby fat. This is the sort of thing that goes on in every part of the body.

THE SHAPE AND HEALTH OF THE BODY DEPENDS ON THE MUSCULAR SYSTEM

Muscles are only too ready to take the line of the least resistance, and do as little work as they can. Often the forearms and upper arms, especially those of women, get flabby in the forties. That, in most cases, is because when using the arms, all the muscles are not being brought into play. Not enough energetic push-and-pull is being put into the movements which are made with the arms.

It does not help matters either, to use hands and arms for work for which they were not intended. Everyday I watch people hauling themselves up from chairs, bus seats, etc., by using their hands and arms ... a job which belongs to the muscles of the diaphragm, abdomen, and thighs. The muscles of the diaphragm, in particular are enormously powerful, or should be. They should not need help from hands or arms in raising the body from the sitting position. The less these muscles are used, the less willing they are to be used, and eventually there comes a time when they are so weak that it is hard manual labor to get out of a chair.

This "helping hand" habit is insidious and very easy to get into without noticing what is happeneing. Before you know where you are, the hands are getting S.O.S. messages from muscles in other parts of the body—from the midriff, legs and thighs, etc. They are being asked to help lower, for instance, the body into a bath (they can legitimately ask for a little help in getting *out* of it); to raise you from a kneeling position, lift you out of bed, and help you into it, and so on.

What we have to aim at, and achieve if we want to make and keep ourselves supple and youthful, is the control of our muscles. That is what I referred to at the beginning of this book as proper organization and control of our muscles. Once that has been done, we have a dynamic force at our command. This force will literally resurrect the body; resurrect it in the dictionary sense of causing "revival from disuse, or inactivity, or decay."

This method of organizing the muscles so that they will obey us is based on a system of muscle control taught by the Greeks in the fifth century. In those days, the Greek race reached a peak of physical perfection which is a byword; even today their beauty is legendary.

These early Greeks knew the importance of the muscular system to bodily health and symmetry. At the age of five, the Greek child began his training at the palaestra (the gymnasium). The child was taught, not muscle development in the usual sense, but the *use* of the muscles. The result aimed at was a muscular condition which achieved perfect co-ordination and control. This made for a mastery of the body and its movements, which few of us today would believe possible. The establishment of correct relationship between muscle and muscle, and their use, meant that fatigue was almost abolished. What we should rate as feats of endurance could be carried out without strain. The secret of achieving this state of co-ordination of the muscles is to establish a condition of tension.

45

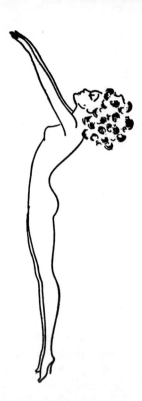

THE NECESSITY OF SPECIALIZED
STRETCHING

Tension in this sense does not mean strain or stress or tenseness. Tension here is used in the sense in which it is used in mechanics, to mean the "pull" which is exercised by and on objects when they are part of a system, either in equilibrium or in motion; which could be loosely translated as "Specialized Stretching." This stretching technique was the basis of Greek physical training.

Scientists have discovered that a muscle in action generates a greater elastic force which produces movement. In a steam-engine, the elastic force of a gas, generated by fuel-combustion, is converted to energy or "work." This is similar to the process which occurs in our living tissues.

One of the effects of achieving the condition of tension is a feeling of lightness - almost a sensation of having overcome the "pull" of gravity which helps to make movement easy and pleasant. This could be because the upward stretch of tension is counteractive to the downward pull of gravity. This downward pull, I believe, affects us more than most of us realize. While we are growing, the upward thrust of life, which operates in all forms of growth, is the stronger force. When we are past maturity, its strength ebbs, unless we have learned how to conserve it. Then, as you might say, the earth begins to reclaim our bodies. We bend, we shrink measurably, we wither; just as a plant withers and returns to the ground, when the life-force which lifted it and enabled it to withstand the drag of gravity, is spent!

When the muscles are in a state of perfect tension, or "weight," the weight of the body is dispersed along their constantly-moving cords, so that no "dead" weight collects at one point, which means that muscle fatigue is almost entirely cut out.

The control center from which this muscular power is generated is the diaphragm. The strength and development of the muscles of the diaphragm condition the rest of the muscular system; it is the center of gravity from which movement radiates. I call the diaphragm "the success muscle." I think the ability to use correctly and to control the diaphragm, gives poise and self-confidence, and is essential to achievement of any kind.

The waist, or middle of the body, is the crucial area. Here are some of the body's most powerful muscles; those of the diaphragm itself, of the abdomen, and the latissima dorsi, the muscles which spread from the spine around each side, forming a natural elastic belt of muscle. In all too many waists, however, there is no sign of these muscles. The condition, instead of tension, is one of chronic crumpling. The slackness of the muscles means that the top half of the body subsides on to the hips, very much like a collapsed concertina. This, more than anything else, produces "middle-aged spread." The pressure of weight of the upper part of the body puts an unnatural strain on the hip muscles. They develop disproportionately, and the hips lose all symmetry. Grecian men and women, as their statues at this period show, had attractively slim hip-lines. You, too, can have a Grecian hip-line when your muscles have learned to work the Greek way.

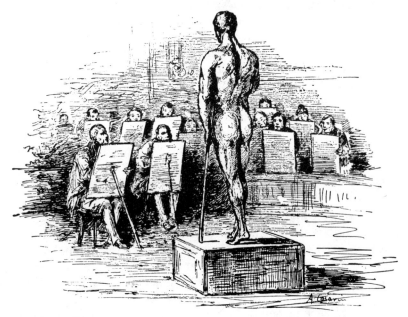

HOW TO DO GREEK SYSTEM OF EXERCISE

What we are going to do is to learn how to produce a condition of tension, or "stretch," in every muscle of the body, including, by the way, the face.

FIRST STEP: Stand in front of a long mirror, with the feet together touching each other. The weight is thrown more forward, on the balls of the feet. The hands are stretched down straight by the sides.

Now check your posture. The old rule of being able to draw an imaginary line from the ear-lobe, through the shoulder, hip-joint and knee, down to the ball of the foot, if you are standing correctly, still holds true. Make sure that you have this right before going on to the next step. If necessary, practice until it comes naturally. It is a waste of time to attempt the rest of the program until you can manage this; you would be likely to use the wrong muscles. Then you would get a condition of tenseness, not tension.

SECOND STEP: Having achieved your correct preliminary posture, draw up from the waist, as if you were trying to pull yourself in two. At the same time, press in the muscles; try to make the front of your waist touch your spine, as it were. This pulling-up action lifts up the rib-cage, and the shoulders go along with it. Be very careful not to raise the shoulders separately, and remember to keep them well pressed back. Stretch downwards with the thighs and legs, so as to exert as much pull against your upward waist movement as possible. Stretch and counter-stretch; that is the principle to keep in mind, and the secret of the success of this method.

THIRD STEP: Now straighten the neck, pulling it up from the shoulders which are pressed back, you will remember. Extend the neck upwards, as much as you can.

FOURTH STEP: Stretch the arms, downwards, as much as you can, and push downwards with each finger, separately. The arm-stretch exerts a counter-stretch against the upward pull of neck and shoulders, but be careful that the shoulders are not dragged downwards.

FIFTH STEP: Against the fulcrum of the stretched and back-pressed neck, push the chin a little forward, and lift it slightly, so that you feel a pull on the muscles under the chin. Now lift the muscles of the face. This is not an easy process to describe, but beginning at the chin, it is possible to raise the muscles of the entire face. If you smile, you will see what I mean. The muscles of the cheeks automatically lift when one

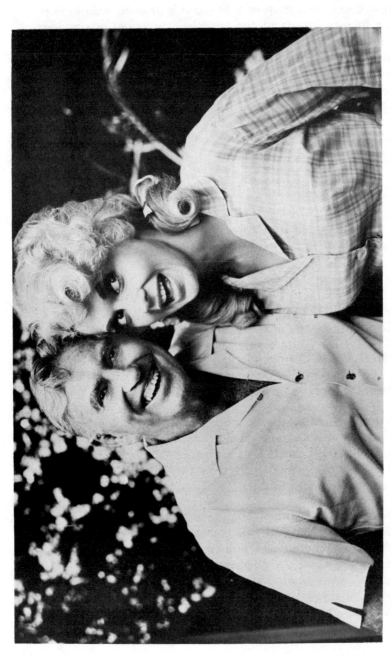

Paul Bragg congratulates Donna Douglas — "Elly May" of the Beverly Hillbillies — not only on her beauty and talent but especially because she is one of the best Health Girls in Hollywood as a result smiles. That is the muscle movement that with practice you can achieve without smiling; a smile is not necessary to this particular excercise. In fact, it is essential not to smile, because the muscles of the mouth have to do their work, and if the lips were parted, different muscles would be brought into play. So you lift the muscles of the face, and the mouth goes with them, held almost in a pout, until the top lip curves up towards the nose. The cheeks lift until the eyes appear almost half-closed. Now open the eyes to their widest extent; raise the eyebrows towards the hairline.

SIXTH STEP: Lastly, brace the muscles of the knee-cap, by pushing the knee-cap back as far as possible. Then rise up on the ball of the toes. The entire body, from the crown of the head to the tips of the toes, is now in a state of tension, and it is well worth practicing until you can achieve that condition. If you find it too difficult to cope with the facial tension, to begin with, as well as that of the body, you can practice the former while sitting down, until you are proficient enough to add it to the general exercise. Remember, you must begin the facial tension with the upward stretch of the diaphragm muscles, and continue with the shoulder, neck and chin movement. A sagging chin begins to sag at the waist; it is a culmination of deterioration of posture and slack muscles of the whole torso.

A NATURAL METHOD OF FACE-LIFTING

When you are practicing "top half" tension, sit erect in a straight-backed chair. Press the end of the spine against the back of the chair, and draw up the spine as much as you can and really draw it up, putting energy in the movement. Try, as in the general excercise, to "pull apart" at the waist, and press in the muscles of the diaphragm and abdomen as hard as you can.

The shoulders, which are lifted by the movement, are pressed well back. Press back the neck, and press the chin a little forward; lift it slightly. Now raise the muscles of the face and chin. Squeeze up the muscles of the cheeks towards the eyes; squeeze up the muscles of the eyes until they appear as slits. Squeeze really hard, without causing strain, of course. Now, against this pressure, try to open the eyes very wide indeed. This exercises and strengthens all the muscles of the face, eyes and neck, as well as those of the waist, diaphragm, and so on.

This is a natural method of dealing with double chins, and crepey necks, and of "face-lifting" in general. The action of the muscles firms and smooths the skin, and reconditions it. Lines under the eyes gradually disappear; the contours of face and neck become firm and youthful again. By the way, I am not describing a beauty treatment which can be skipped by men. The muscles of the face, neck and eyes are as important, in their way, as those of the rest of the body. They must be kept in trim and fit by anyone who wants to realize a condition of complete Health and Internal Fitness.

As the diaphragm is the control center of the operation of tension, and as the strengthening of its muscles is a pre-requisite of achieving that condition, it is a good plan to practice as often as possible the "stretching" of the diaphragm, pulling the waist up and pressing it in. Apart from its benefits to Health and Internal Fitness (firm muscles support the vital organs), this movement results in a slim, trim, supple waist, and acts as a hip-reducer. This stretching is one the exercises used by Spanish dancers; you may have noticed their slender waists and hips. Many of them spend regular periods each day with arms lifted high above their heads, trying to reach the ceiling, pulling up the body strongly from the waist. You can do this, too, if you wish. It is a way of speeding up results, and a great aid to figure-beauty.

It was through watching Spanish dancers, Indian women water-carriers, and a Mexican dancer that I realized what the principle of "stretching" correctly applied, can do for the human body in the promotion of Health, Internal Fitness and Symmetry! It can produce, as I have just mentioned, lovely trim and fit lines of waist and hip. It makes the necks of the Indian women who carried heavy earthenware Chatthis (vessels) of water on their heads smooth and firm, even when the women were very old. It made the hands and arms of the Mexican woman dancer who stretched and turned and twisted these parts of her body daily white and smooth and supple as those of a twenty-year-old, although her age was sixty.

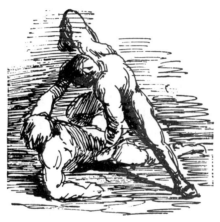

DEFENSE AGAINST PREMATURE AGEING

The principle of stretching can be used on any part of the body to preserve and to help restore youth. But to get the best results, the condition of complete tension must be achieved. I have described the "sitting stretch," which is one of the ways of getting the muscles into practice for this condition. Another is the arm and leg stretch. The best place to do this is in the bath, because then the muscles are relaxed. When in that state they carry out, with less effort, demands made on them.

Sit up straight, with the spine pressed against the back of the bath, and stretch the spine as much as possible - gently, of course. Never let an opportunity go by for exercising this all-important part of your body - the spine. A straight, supple spine is a strong defense against premature ageing; it is your life-line!

Having got your spine into position with particular care that the "small" of your back makes contact with the back of the bath, make sure that the diaphragm is drawn well up and in. During the whole exercise, the diaphragm must be kept in that position; the shoulders must be pressed well back, and the buttocks pressed against the bath.

Now lift the left leg at an angle of about 75 degrees to the body. Stretch as if you were trying to disengage it from the hip socket. The stretch must bring the muscles of the entire leg into play; press back the knee-cap, stretch the calf muscles; stretch the foot, and without moving the ankle, try to bend the foot downwards as far as possible, from the instep. Do not strain. After a moment drop the left leg, and repeat with the right leg. Then lift the left leg at the same angle as before, and again stretch in the same way, but this time try to bend the foot at the instep over towards you. After a minute or two, relax, and repeat with the right leg.

Now, still keeping the same position against the back of the bath, and with the diaphragm well squeezed in, lift your left arm. The shoulders must be kept firmly against the bath, acting as a fulcrum to the stretching process, which is carried out by extending the left arm. hand and fingers (which must be kept touching), as fully as you can, in front of you. The stretch must be felt in each finger-tip. Without moving the shoulder, turn the arm inside out, so to speak, so that the palm of the hand and the inside of the elbow, are facing you. Keep turning until the movement becomes uncomfortable - but do not strain. Then relax and then repeat with the right arm. Now extend the left arm, as before. This time, turn the arm so that the palm of the hand is turned away from you. When you can turn the arm no farther, relax. Repeat with the right arm.

This is what one could call a "muscle reveille." It wakes up lazy muscles, and, incidentally, limbers up the joints. Don't forget full extension and stretching of the fingers. At the end of this exercise, double up the fingers, and press them hard against the palms of the hands, with the thumb folded over the bent fingers. Squeeze fingers and thumbs hard. You can do this finger and hand stretching and clenching whenever you have a spare moment. It is a great help towards keeping the hands supple, flexible, and healthy—and very youthful looking. Your hands tell how old you are.

And before we leave the bath, a word about how to leave it. Don't depend on the hands and arms to do all the lifting of your body from the water. They will have to do a little of the work, but practice lifting and squeezing the diaphragm muscles, and put them and the abdominal and thigh muscles to work on the lifting job. Do not strain ever. As the muscles strengthen, you will find that you are able to get up more and more easily, until finally a slight push with the hands against the sides of the bath is all that is necessary in the way of assistance.

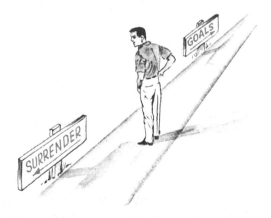

"IF AT FIRST YOU DON'T SUCCEED . . . "

Do not be discouraged if at first your muscles show no sign of obeying you. Usually, once they have been allowed to get lazy, they are opposed to going back to work. They send messages of despair to the brain: "It's quite impossible. This movement can never be done. We are too weak and our bones are too stiff."

Do not believe them. If you will keep on practicing, day after day, eventually the movement that you thought out of the question will just seem to happen. The body has almost illimitable powers of response; most of us never even tap these powers. Let me tell you of a case of a woman who did make use of these possibilities.

She was a very prematurely old woman of seventy-two; terribly out of shape physically. Every muscle in her body was weak and flabby. She had very little endurance and stamina. She was as stiff as a board. Every muscle and joint seemed to be cemented. Then she told me that she wished to take up swimming and diving. She could not swim one stroke. In fact, all her life she was terribly afraid of the water. But she thought swimming and diving would be helpful in reconditioning her stiff shoulders, neck, arms, hips, knees and feet.

But she had a strong desire to achieve something and that is all that counts! The mind can make a weak body rejuvenate itself. Flesh is dumb . . . the mind must rule the flesh.

I put her on a natural eating program, gave her the correct food supplements and put her to work on the "Tension Exercises." In three months she started her swimming and diving lessons. In one year it was remarkable how well she swam and dived. A triumph of mind over matter. But she found the trouble she had taken well worthwhile. She said that her muscles and the joints of her legs, hands, thighs, and hips had become supple again, and that her general health was perfect.

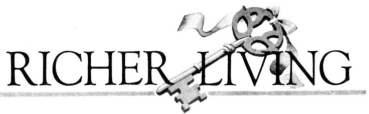

RICHER LIVING

IT IS NEVER TOO LATE TO GET INTERNAL PHYSICAL FITNESS

At first you will be awkward, stiff and sore from your "tension" exercises. But that will last only a short time. As you build up a good circulation, your muscles will begin to strengthen, and obey you. You will discover how comfortable this condition of stretch or tension is. Your body, instead of being about as manageable as a sack of potatoes, (as are most bodies with flabby and untrained muscular systems), is under the control of your will. Movement begins to be a pleasure instead of a wearisome, and perhaps painful, process. You actually feel you want to move for the sheer pleasure of it, for the sense of well-being it produces. And that feeling is not illusory; it is real. Movement of the right kind stimulates glandular secretions. So you feel better, and you are better, and you want to use the body more and more. The body was made for use; so a circle, not of the vicious, but of the constructive type, is formed.

You must be very conscious of your diaphragm and keep it pulled in. Get that feeling that your tummy is touching your backbone. Don't lean on anything when standing—make your muscles support your body at all times. And when you want to sit—*DO NOT CROSS YOUR LEGS*. Look at the men and women who make a constant habit of crossing the legs when they sit down and you will find the veins and blood vessels of the legs are deteriorating. The circulation must flow through the body with ease. When you sit with the *LEGS CROSSED*, you are shutting off over 75% of the circulation going into the legs. The heart is having a hard enough time of circulating the blood through the arteries and veins without your *CROSS-ING THE LEGS* and making the heart work that much harder.

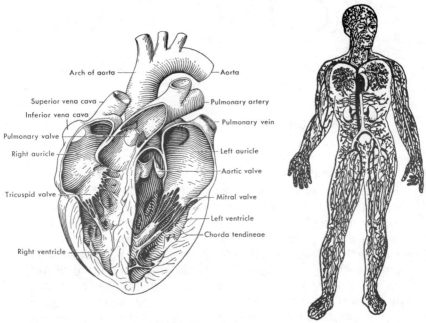

The heart is really a double pump, each side composed of two chambers, an auricle and a ventricle.

Circulatory system. Showing arteries and veins.

THE HEART - THE STRONGEST MUSCLE IN THE BODY

It has been estimated that some 40% of all people over forty years of age have a significant degree of obstructions owing to hardening of the arteries and veins. Therefore, they are candidates for some kind of heart problems. Your heart has a tremendous job to do to keep you on top of this earth. Simply described, the heart is a pump. It pumps about 2000 gallons of blood every 24 hours. An average heart pumps 70 times to the minute; with strenuous exertion it may pump 120 times a minute. In an average life-span of 70 years it pumps 2½ billion times. It is the most wonderful pump ever designed and is about as big as your fist. The chief function of the heart is to pump blood to all parts of the body. The blood is pumped through vessels to circulate and recirculate in a continuous process. To do this pumping work, the muscles of the heart itself need a constant supply of energy and nourishment. They get this supply from oxygen and certain nutrients carried in the blood. Blood is specially channeled to the heart by its own network of arteries known as the coronary arteries.

The heart cannot function without a proper supply of blood, and it never functions well if the blood-supply is restricted.

Restriction of the blood-supply through the coronary artery system may be caused by hardening of the arteries (arteriosclerosis). It may be caused by a narrowing of the bore of the arteries owing to deposits of fat and other material on the inside lining of the arteries, much as the pipes from a kitchen sink may become narrowed by a continual depositing of waste material.

Hardening of the arteries, plus this depositing of fatty material inside the vessels, resulting in a narrowing of the passage through the vessels, thus restricts the flow of blood to the heart.

That is the reason we must be active people. The more we exercise and keep active, the more we pump blood through the arteries and keep the arteries flexible and the passages open.

Let's review some of the principles of a Physically Fit existence. These can be considered guidelines that you should follow for the rest of your life.

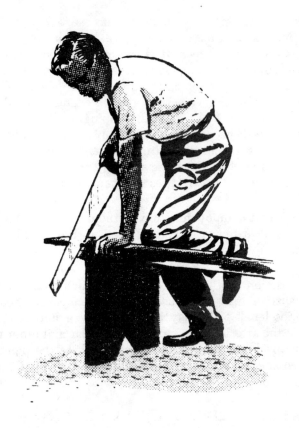

LET'S BUILD A STRONG HEART

Keep active! Don't be a sitter! Walk, walk, walk! Climb stairs! Swim! Dance, run, jog, skip! Exercise! Do everything you can to promote the flow of your blood through the circulatory system, to open up capillaries (the small pipes of the body) which might otherwise stay unopened, in order to strengthen the heart and improve the function of the blood vessels. As a result, your pulse rate will remain slow, the stroke volume of your heart will remain sharp and strong.

You should take cold baths. Don't let the flabby weakling frighten you by saying that cold water is a shock to the heart and the nervous system. Cold bathing is a great aid to maintain good muscular tone and circulatory and respiratory fitness, and to keep down nervous tension. The stimulation of cool water on the skin produces a mild vaso-constriction which forces the blood inward and increases its supply to the inner organs, the glands, the heart and the nerve centers. Once you've gotten used to the mild shock of cold water, you'll find your cold bath a calming and refreshing experience. Outdoor activity, including moderate exposure to wind, sun and cold, should be part of your year-round activity.

Don't be a hot-house plant. Condition yourself to take any kind of weather. Let the weaklings worry about drafts, chills, wet feet and all the other things the weaklings fear. Build up a good vigorous constitution.

Your body can be built into a powerhouse of energy and vitality, but it will never be handed to you on a silver-platter. All the good things of life, including perfect Internal Physical Fitness, have to be earned. There is no easy system to health and long life.

You have to eat plenty of raw fruits and vegetables. Give your digestive system a 24-hour rest once a week by eating nothing; that is, by fasting with nothing passing through your system but pure water (preferably distilled water).

Your diet should be supplemented with an adequate amount of minerals and vitamins. When you take food supplements, you are assured of getting the important vitamins, minerals, and nutrients your body needs.

Every morning make a Health Cocktail of two teaspoons of natural cider vinegar and one or two teaspoons of honey with water added. At least 6 ounces of water. Pure natural apple cider vinegar and honey give the body many important nutrients. You will see and feel the benefits of this Health Cocktail!

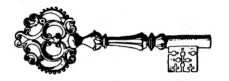

A STRICT PROGRAM OF MIND CONTROL,

VIGOROUS EXERCISE AND NATURAL

EATING PAYS OFF WITH MORE

HEALTH AND ENERGY

Your mind must control your body. It is a sad fact that most people are controlled by their bodies.

FLESH IS DUMB! You can put any food rubbish in your body: hot dogs, pizza pies, cremated hamburgers, cakes, candy, salted nuts, salted potato chips, fried foods, salty foods, sugared foods, rich, gooey pastries, etc. You can wash this trash down with coffee, tea, beer, cola drinks, soft drinks - flesh is dumb and will accept any abuse you give it. Only an intelligent mind with wisdom and knowledge can discipline the body. Mind over matter is the important rule to follow. Your mind must rule every cell and organ in your body.

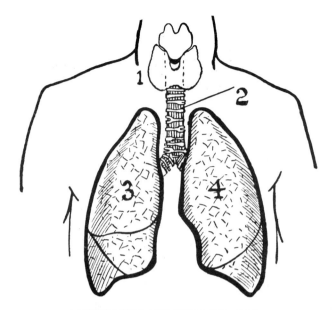

THE LUNGS AND THE WINDPIPE

(1) Thyroid Gland in front of (2) Windpipe,
(3) and (4) Right and Left Lungs.

EVERY MORNING DO YOUR POSTURE EXERCISE YOUR STRETCHING EXERCISES AND FULL DEEP BREATHING

Your body needs oxygen and the only way you can get this invisible nutrient is through full deep breathing. You must make it a daily habit to do forced deep-breathing exercises. Just pucker your mouth as if you were going to whistle. Now draw the air in the lungs and at the same time expand the diaphragm. Remember, I have stated that the diaphragm is the key to vitality and great strength. With each full breath push the diaphragm out. Pretend that you have a tummy full of air (which is what you have). Hold the breath for three seconds and then force the air out of the body with great effort, drawing in the diaphragm. Draw in the tummy until you feel as if it is touching the backbone.

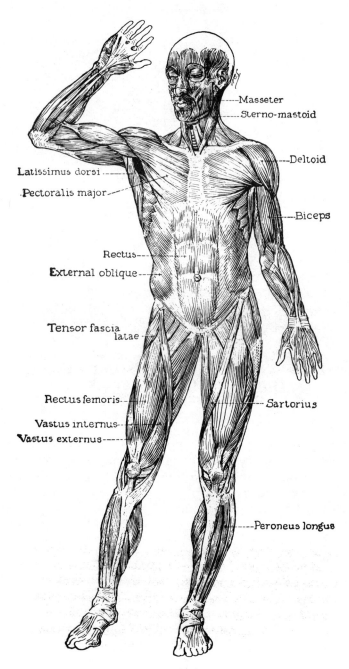

Masseter
Sterno-mastoid

Deltoid

Latissimus dorsi

Pectoralis major

Biceps

Rectus

External oblique

Tensor fascia
latae

Rectus femoris

Sartorius

Vastus internus
Vastus externus

Peroneus longus

64

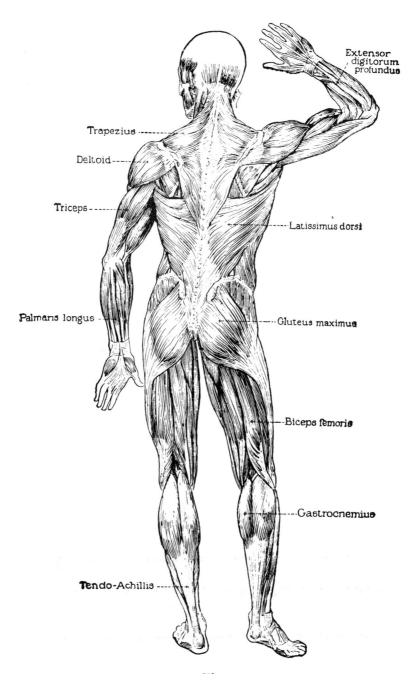

Extensor digitorum profundus

Trapezius

Deltoid

Triceps

Palmaris longus

Latissimus dorsi

Gluteus maximus

Biceps femoris

Gastrocnemius

Tendo-Achillis

During the day whenever you think of it, draw the tummy in and make it touch your backbone. Be conscious that you have a diaphragm. Educate it and work it! You will be filled with vitality every waking hour of the day. Once you start your Internal Fitness program stick to it rigidly, for you will find if you succumb to the temptation to skip a day or two, it will be more difficult to resume exercising, postural exercises and full diaphragm breathing the following day. So stick rigidly to your schedule. Any puddin'-head can stay in bed; it takes a person with character and internal strength to get up early enough every morning to take care of and exercise this wonderful body that the Creator has given him.

GOOD AND BAD WAYS TO:

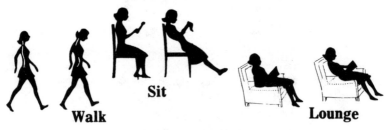

Walk **Sit** **Lounge**

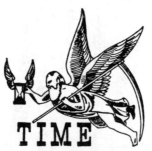

I have just a little minute,
Only sixty seconds in it,
Just a tiny little minute,
Give account if I abuse it;
Forced upon me; can't refuse it.
Didn't seek it, didn't choose it,
But it's up to me to use it.
I must suffer if I lose it;
But eternity is in it.—Unknown.

THE ONE, THE ONLY PERFECT EXERCISE—
THIS IT IT—THE BEST!

   This exercise stretches nearly every one of the six hundred or more muscles of the body. Stand with your legs apart. Swing your right arm up and overhead counter-clockwise across body, then bend from the waist with knees stiff and touch (or try to touch) your left big toe. You won't do it

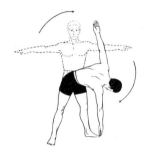

the first time, but stretch down as far as you can. When your back becomes more supple, you will easily touch your left big toe. Then whip arm back overhead, fast and hard, and bend backwards from the waist. All this should, of course, be one continuous movement. Now repeat, using left arm. Swing left arm up and overhead, bend and try to touch

the right big toe. While doing this exercise, suck in and blow out air forcefully, exhaling while touching the toe and inhaling while changing sides. Do the exercise 10 times.

ONE OF THE GREATEST EXERCISES
FOR CIRCULATION

Standing upright, swing both your arms across the front

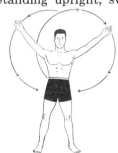

of your body in the opposite direction from each other, up and down in full arm circles. Rhythmically rise on the balls of your feet with each upward swing of the arms, taking regular, full deep breaths, inhaling as you swing the arms up, exhaling as you swing the arms down.

ONE OF THE OLDEST EXERCISES KNOWN TO MAN AND STILL ONE OF THE BEST

This exercise keeps you supple and flexible . . . stand with toes and heels together, keeping legs together and your knees locked. Raise both hands overhead and stretch them as high as you can. Draw in the diaphragm so it touches your spine (or rather feels that way). Bend at the waist, keeping the knees stiff, and try to touch your toes with your fingertips, but don't strain. You must keep practicing and soon you will touch your toes easily. Exhale as you bend down toward your toes and inhale as you come back to starting position. Do exercise 15 times.

EXERCISE FOR IMPROVING YOUR BALANCE

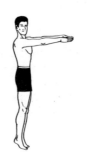

Stand up on your toes, with your heels together, your eyes closed, and your arms stretched forward at the shoulders. Stay in this position for 20 seconds without shifting your feet or opening your eyes. Do this exercise 10 times.

EXERCISES FOR THE SIDE MUSCLES OF THE BODY— THESE MUSCLES ARE KNOWN AS THE BINDING MUSCLES—THEY HELP KEEP YOUR WAIST TRIM, SLIM AND FIRM!

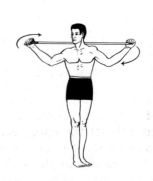

Hold a broomstick behind your neck and shoulders; swing left and right as many times as you can from the waist. Start with ten movements right and left.

STRENGTH-BUILDING EXERCISE FOR HANDS, ARMS, SHOULDERS, BACK, LEGS, ANKLES AND FEET

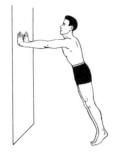

Facing the wall, with your feet placed about thirty or more inches away, lean forward with your hands on the wall, so that the wall is holding you up. Then push up and on your toes and press from toes up through body to hand on the wall. You can also do wall push-ups in this position, where you bend elbows and touch chin to wall.

THE GREATEST EXERCISE FOR STRENGTHENING THE LOWER ABDOMINAL MUSCLES AND THE LOWER SPINE

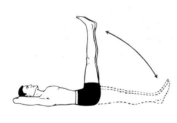

Starting Position: Lie on back with hands clasped behind neck. The Exercise: Holding legs together, raise them to a vertical position, then lower slowly to the floor. Start doing this exercise 5 times, and add more repetitions as your abdomen and spine get stronger.

TORSO ROTATION FOR STRENGTHENING WAIST MUSCLES

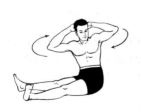

Starting Position: Sit on the floor, with legs extended to the front and both hands clasped behind neck. The Exercise: Twist the upper part of your body to the left as far as you can, then rotate to the right. Do this exercise ten twists on each side.

EXERCISES FOR SLIMMING AND TRIMMING THE HIPS

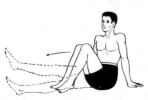

Starting Position: Sit with hands on floor beside hips, with legs extended. The Exercise: Draw both legs up together until your heels are almost touching your buttocks, then thrust them out to extended position. Do this exercise 10 times — do more as your strength increases.

EXERCISE FOR STRENGTHENING THIGHS, ABDOMEN AND BACK

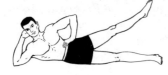

Staring Position: Lie on the right side, with left hand on left hip and right hand supporting head. The Exercise: Raise left leg up and down in rapid whipping motion. Do fifteen times on each side.

BACK STRAIGHTENER EXERCISE

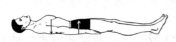

Starting Position: Lie flat on back, with arms at side. The Exercise: Take a big long full breath, and flatten the lower part of your back to the floor for five seconds, then relax. Repeat 7 times, exhaling fully with release.

THESE EXERCISES ARE GOOD FOR BOTH
MEN AND WOMEN

My program for Internal Physical Fitness applies equally to men and women. In fact, in some respects the message of this book applies even more strongly to women than it does to men.

Women, as a rule, are more conscious of their physical beings than men are. They are more sensitive to the ageing process, and naturally want to hold on to their youthful beauty and vitality, and retain a good figure and a clear, fresh youthful and attractive complexion. For this reason, they will go to greater efforts to help themselves than most men will.

But in this country, women are very poorly educated in the scientific facts about physical fitness and how to obtain natural beauty from within! They are brain-washed by advertising and publicity urging them to dye their hair, spend hours upon hours in beauty parlors getting beauty treatments, etc. . . . all of this to frantically try to remain youthful and beautiful!

They are made to believe that beauty and attractiveness come from the outside in. The more creams and lotions they put on their faces, the prettier they will be. Now, cosmetics are very necessary for helping keep the skin clean and moisturized, but creams are not the full answer to the way to keep youthful looking. Cosmetics have their rightful place in a beauty program. But, good natural diet and exercise are what I call "internal cosmetics." No vibrating machine can tighten the facial muscles like exercise which will remove ugly fat and fat spots.

For over 50 years I have been Diet Advisor and Physical Conditioner to some of the highest paid movie stars, T.V. Stars and actresses in Hollywood. I try to explain to these women that youthful vigor and beauty, good complexion, and a trim but vigorous body can come only from the inside. It is a combination of good natural diet exercise, and a program of deep breathing that will make them beautiful and keep them youthful for many, many years.

Some women shy away from physical fitness programs with the wrong psychological attitude that there is something unfeminine about vigorous exercising of the muscles. I want to impress on every woman the fact that there is absolutely no adequate substitute for planned exercise, walking in the fresh air, swimming and running, no matter what the glamor advertisements may say.

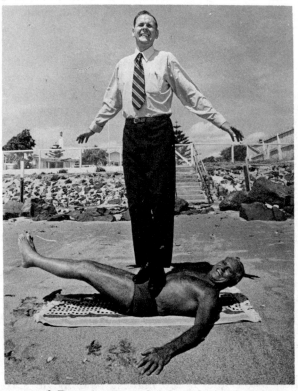

Every part of Bragg's powerful body is fit. He has strong, powerful muscles. Yes even his stomach muscles are strong — for here he is shown with a six foot man standing on his stomach at Milford Beach near Auckland, New Zealand,

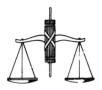

THE NATURAL SYSTEM NEVER FAILS

I know the science of Physical Culture and Nutrition, and with these tools to work with, I can take any woman - young, middle-aged or down-right old - and with her desire and cooperation to beautify herself, I can transform her into a thing of beauty. Any woman who will follow this program of instruction will soon see what natural diet and exercise will do for her.

Last year I took a 68-year old woman who was prematurely old, flabby and out of condition, and put her through this course of instructions. In a little over 11 months of this Internal Fitness program she transformed herself to a thing of beauty. She improved her skin and muscle tone, enriched her blood with good natural diet, and made herself into an attractive woman of whom any woman would be proud. (I attended her wedding a short time ago to a man of 60.)

This course of instruction is keyed to build energy and vitality. A youthful figure isn't worth much without a youthful vigorousness to go with it.

Natural diet and exercise will not only help a woman look more youthful and attractive—it will also make her realize that most women exist in a low scale of health. They are great complainers of their health. They are great pill takers. So, if you are a woman, you can follow the instructions given in this book. You may have to go a little slowly at first until you can condition your muscles to vigorous exercise—but once you have worked the soreness out of your muscles you will show improvement fast. All it takes is a back-bone instead of a wish-bone. It takes a little imagination and plenty of will power.

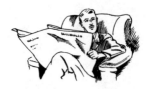

WHAT ABOUT THE AVERAGE MAN?

And this all goes for the men too. Men who are out of shape physically can really create a miracle in their bodies by following this natural system of rejuvenation. Most men when they reach their forties are really on the downgrade physically. They huff and puff at the slightest effort. Their hips get flabby and they develop a sagging pouch. Their legs get weak, and they have little stamina. They tire easily and depend on coffee, tea, tobacco, alcohol and stimulants to keep them going. They over-work. They get full of stress, strains and tensions. They smoke, and that really damages the arteries, heart, lungs and lowers their endurance.

I belong to many men's clubs—and it is really shocking how many die long before their time. But if they *do* exist, they are only half-men. Work, success, business, making money are all very well—but there is something more in life than these things. Without Health, Strength and Vitality all the rest is simply mud.

I have proven to hundreds of men that they can be a success in the world—and still have a youthful, internally fit body, regardless of age. If men will give this program their whole-hearted support, they could make new people out of themselves.

The recuperative powers of man's body are tremendous. All you have to do is to be determined that you will work with nature by eating correctly and by exercising the muscles of the body.

It's a simple system—all honest truthful things are simple. Nature intended it to be that way.

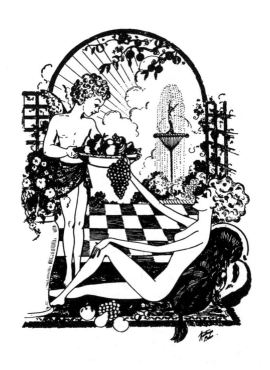

FOOD: THE BASIC FACTOR OF LIFE

Every activity of mind and the body depends in greater or in lesser extent upon the food we eat. In that sense, food is the basic factor of our lives, and nutrition is the basic science. The wrong food can be a destructive influence, causing illness, affecting mental powers, shortening life. The right food can be a safeguard against ill-health; can build us up on all levels and, we have seen, can make a powerful contribution towards long life and long youth.

Yet almost nothing is known about eating, generally; about eating in its real sense, I mean. And this always seems to be a blind-spot in the human race. Would you turn a child, who knew only the ABC of chemistry, loose in a laboratory stocked with powerful chemicals, some of them dangerous, and let him play about with them, just as he fancied? He could, with no trouble at all, blow himself up, or burn or mutilate himself. He would be lucky to escape without some form of injury. Yet when most of us sit down to lunch, or dinner, in our lack of knowledge of the effects on our system of what we are putting into our stomachs, we are very much in the same boat as the child in the laboratory. The effects of food chemicals may not be so spectacular or so immediate as those in the laboratory, but they are just as certain. They are governed by the laws of biochemistry.

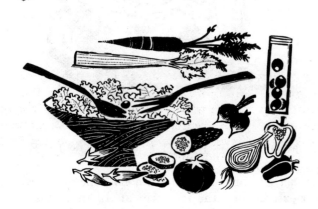

COMMON-SENSE NUTRITION

The common-sense thing, you would think, would be to have elementary facts of nutrition taught in all schools, but not by the dictates of the commercial food processor as it is today. Today a person like myself who believes in natural scientific nutrition would not be allowed to teach in any school.

Why? Because everything made of bleached white flour, refined white sugar, white rice, hot dogs, lunch meats, processed cheese, cola drinks, packaged mashed potatoes, deep fried potatoes would be thrown out of the instruction on feeding. That would hurt the food processor where it hurts the most—his bank-account. There is not a chance today for a child or an adult, for that matter, to learn natural scientific nutrition. The idiot box, the T.V., is brain-washing all Americans to eat the foodless foods that are produced by the food processor.

But, if it were possible to give the children and the adults the truth about eating, what a difference we should see in our national health in just one generation. Centers where facts are available could be established in every city and village in the country. Some way should be found to get across vital, practical information about the right use of food, to adults— men as well as women. And it should be found without delay, before the standard of national health drops any lower. People constantly ask me why no such places exist; it is one of my dreams to see such centers come into being: centers where people could be shown the vital relationship between food and health and youth and long life ... where mothers would discover why Jane can't eat eggs, or why Willie doesn't like vegetables. Childish likes and dislikes of certain foods may seem trivial, but often they are valuable clues to the body's workings. They can be followed up, used to safeguard health, to improve "difficult" characters (which often are due to dietary deficiencies), and even make schoolwork easier, by increasing mental ability and aiding memory.

To bring all this about, the average person need not get bogged down with a lot of complicated detail; it would be enough to know the broad principles of Natural Scientific Nutrition, just what I am giving in this course of instruction.

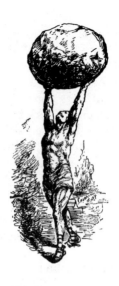

THIS IS THE IDEAL DIET FOR
BUILDING HEALTH

I want you to make 50 to 70 percent of your diet raw fruits and vegetables and properly cooked fruits and vegetables; to eat only 100% natural stone ground whole grains for bread and cereals; to eat lean meat not more than three times a week, if you desire meat as your protein. Fish, in my opinion, is better than meat as a protein because it is so low in saturated fats. You can have four eggs per week, you can have sunflower seeds, sesame seeds, all kinds of nuts and nut butters, soya beans, lentils, and the various dried bean including the garbanzas which are a good food. You should use the natural unsaturated oils for your salads and cooking such as safflower oil, olive oil, corn oil, etc.; you should use brown rice instead of the white polished rice. There are over two hundred items a person can eat that are delicious and nutritious and are classed as good nutrition. In other words, you could, this very minute, make out a perfectly balanced meal program for yourself for a week from what I just told you. Let me show you how it is done.

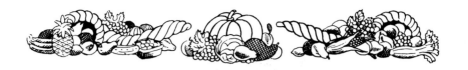

A SAMPLE DAY'S PROGRAM FOR A
BALANCED DIET

Morning program:

After your exercises - A HEALTH COCKTAIL

1 tsp. pure apple cider vinegar or juice of ½ lemon
1 tsp. pure natural honey
1 cup water (warm if desired) preferably distilled water

This health cocktail is the very best you can take because it is rich in natural acids that your body uses for internal cleansing, and it is a rich source of potassium which the body needs for complete functioning.

BREAKFAST: A large dish of prunes with plenty of liquid.

Here's how I prepare my prunes: Soak one pound of prunes over-night in one quart of water to which a washed, sliced orange has been added, skin and all. In the morning you can eat them just as they are. If you do apply heat, do it this way so that you do not destroy the nutrients. Put them on the fire and bring them to a boil. Then shut off the heat at once and allow to cool before eating. They will keep in the refrigerator for several days. On these prunes use from 1 to 7 teaspoons of raw wheat germ and sweeten with honey.

1 egg (a hard boiled egg is the best nutritional way to eat an egg, I have found in my researches. No grease is necessary in its preparation). If you wish toast, be sure it is made of 100% whole grains. I believe that rye and corn bread are the best grains we can use. I have made many tests with whole-grains but these grains, in my opinion, have the greatest amount of value to the body.

If you desire a warm drink, there are many delicious herb beverages such as Mint Tea, Alfalfa-Mint Tea, and many others from your Health Food Store. Don't snack between meals. It is a bad habit. Give the digestive organs a chance to digest your meal before you start putting more food into your body. You may have fresh fruit between meals, or a small drink of fruit or vegetable juice.

LUNCH:

Lunch time should be salad time. A raw vegetable combination is the very best thing you can eat from a nutritional stand-point. You can have a salad dressing of pure cider vinegar and some unsaturated oil or lemon juice and oil. At lunch you should not eat protein if you expect to go back to work and feel wide-awake and alert. Your combination salad and several cooked vegetables will send you back to work with mental and physical alertness and let you escape the later afternoon period of drowsiness or low energy. In the afternoon, if you desire, you may have fresh fruit or a small glass of fresh fruit or vegetable juice.

DINNER:

This should be the important meal of the day. The tensions, stress and strains are over. The rushing is over. It is now time to sit down to a wholesome nutritious meal. It should be a happy meal. Joyfulness is good for the digestion. We at our home make the evening meal gay and festive. We play our favorite music and most of the time eat by soft candlelight. (Even when I eat alone in the evening I do the same as when I am with the family and friends.) We always start our meals with a fresh raw vegetable salad.

SUGGESTED DINNER:

Cole Slaw (Made from crisp fresh green cabbage, chilled, shredded and tossed).

Health mayonnaise dressing.

Celery and carrot sticks.

Protein of your selection which could be lean meat, (no pork), fish, or poultry. (Or you may select a vegetarian protein: soya beans, lentils, garbanzas-called chick beans by many, lima beans, pinto beans, kidney beans or brown rice.)

Nuts provide you with another fine source of protein. Almonds, with skins on (unblanched) are one of the best. Pecans, walnuts, nuts, hazel nuts are all good natural protein foods. Sunflower seeds, pumpkin seeds and sesame seeds are rich in protein. Twice a week, but no more, you could use a natural cheese for your protein, if you desire. Remember all dairy products are mucus-forming and contain a great amount of cholesterol which sometimes blocks the circulatory system of the body. Go very lightly on the dairy products.

Avocados are a splendid source of protein with their wonderful unsaturated fat.

DESSERT:

I think this is a habit that should be eliminated from all meals, as it tends to over-eating. When you have eaten a substantial, wholesome meal, why stuff something extra into the stomach to overwork it? If you *must* have something for dessert, have a baked apple, or apple sauce. These should be sweetened with honey; never eat any food with white sugar.

Make your eating simple. Eat all food as close to its original state as possible—that is, as fresh as you can get it. Keep away from fancy packaged good. These foods must have a long shelf life and, in order to have this, all the perishable part of the food is manufactured out of it. Look at the labels on all foods you eat and when they say sugar, keep away from them. Such foods as lunch meats, sausages, and hot dogs have all been chemically preserved. Keep them out of your stomach. Ice cream, white rice, soft and cola drinks, jams, jellies, pastries form no part of our Internal Fitness program.

NOTE: You should have my *Bragg Health Food Cook Book* to give you full instructions for preparing perfect keep-fit meals. (See Back Cover.)

Remember, you are what you eat. You can either eat yourself to illness and an early grave or you can eat your way to Internal Physical Fitness which will give you a long, happy, healthy life.

Ponce de Leon,

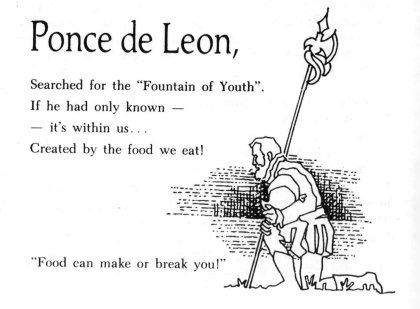

Searched for the "Fountain of Youth".

If he had only known —

— it's within us...

Created by the food we eat!

"Food can make or break you!"

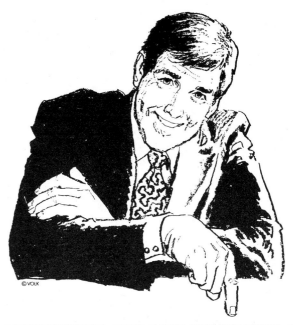

ADVERTISING OUR LOW STANDARDS OF HEALTH

When next you are in a bus, or reading a newspaper or magazine or watching T.V. or listening to the radio, notice the advertisements, and you will see what I mean about the national health standard. I haven't actually worked out the proportion of different types of advertisements, but I think there's no doubt that those concerned with remedies for illness of some kind are far ahead numerically of any of the others. Headaches, colds, coughs, fatigue, constipation, indigestion, overweight, wherever we go, we can't escape from reminders that most of us sputter, wheeze, hiccup, belch our way through life, and stumble along with stiff joints, aching backs and are racked by rheumatism or arthritis. Food is not the panacea for all this—please don't misunderstand me as saying that. But it is, I repeat, the basic factor, and we should give it the attention which it deserves. It is good balanced nutrition, vigorous exercise, deep breathing, sound restful sleep and a tranquil mind that combine to give Internal Physical Fitness.

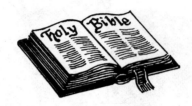

Man cannot live by bread alone. Each one of us must put our faith and our trust in a Power higher than ourselves. We must have spiritual food also. We must have faith in something far above ourselves to keep us going in this cruel world. Throughout my life, the 23rd Psalm has been the firm rock that has helped me every day of my life:

The Lord is my shepherd; I shall not want.
He maketh me to lie down in green pastures: He leadeth me beside the still waters.
He restoreth my soul: He leadeth me in the paths of righteousness for His name's sake.
Yea, though I walk through the valley of the shadow of death, I will fear no evil:
for Thou art with me; Thy rod and Thy staff they comfort me.
Thou preparest a table before me in the presence of mine enemies: Thou anointest my head with oil; my cup runneth over.
Surely goodness and mercy shall follow me all the days of my life; and I will dwell in the house of the Lord forever.

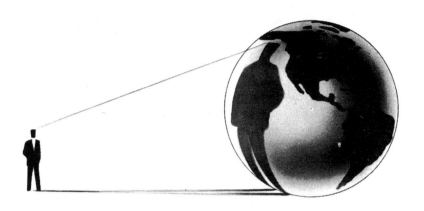

WE MUST CONSIDER MAN:
BODY, MIND AND SPIRIT

We must consider man: body, mind and spirit. We must develop ourselves on all these planes of living. Therefore, spiritual food is necessary to the body. There are many kinds of religions and faiths; there are many soul-lifting philosophies that we can go to for mental and spiritual strength. I believe that the closest thing to God is your conscience. There, I think, a soft voice can help you go in the right direction. I try in my daily life to listen to this voice for guidance.

I have a meditation period twice daily, in the morning and before retiring, where I contact the God-head in my body. I seek help and guidance from this Higher Power. I find it gives not only spiritual strength but it gives me the will power to carry out my program of Internal Physical Fitness.

I feel a companionship with God and Nature. I feel the great strength these powers give me as I am working with forces higher than myself. I am getting strength from the Infinite . . . this Power is all about us; it is an invisible Power that you can contact. It is Power that can give a reason for living. It can give you confidence. When I exercise I call on this invisible Power to give me energy. I know that when I eat natural food, especially raw fruits and vegetables, I am contacting it. When I hike, run, swim, play, I let this infinite Power flow through me. Let me explain how powerful a force this is, and how you can draw upon it.

Three small boys went out into the forest for a hike. A sudden storm broke and a little boy got pinned under a falling tree. It was a brutually heavy tree. When the other two boys saw the disaster that had happened to their friend, they tried to lift the heavy log from the helpless boy. With superhuman strength they succeeded and saved the boy's life.

The next day the boys who lifted the tree brought their fathers and friends to see the enormous tree they had raised. They tried to lift the tree again, the fathers and friends helping, but with all their combined strength they could not lift the tree one inch from the ground. Originally, however, those boys had done it alone. In their hour of crisis, they had this Power of which I am speaking.

People ask me how I can swim long distances in rough sea water without fear of drowning. It's hard to explain to them that it is not only my own body strength that allows me to swim long distances, but that when I am in the water I am using this infinite Power of the universe. It is everywhere . . . cosmic energy. We can draw upon it. The cleaner, the purer our bodies get through natural living, the closer to nature we get, the more we can have of this unlimited cosmic Power. Become a child of nature and many wonderful experiences will happen to you.

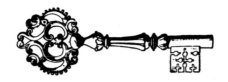

THE POWER OF THE GOLDEN KEY

When you are working with nature by exercising and eating natural food, you make your body a powerful receiving instrument for great universal power. That is the reason I fast one 24-hour period every week, and from seven to ten days at every new season. As I write these very lines to you, I am in my eighth day of fasting. You think I would be weak—but I have been at my typewriter for hours and in a short time I am going out for my daily long swim, a run and a hike and sunbathing. Power is flowing in my clean body. I feel a surge of powerful energy in body, mind and spirit. I am in tune with the Infinite. I am one with Nature. My powers of concentration are great; I have peace of mind and I am in harmony with God and Nature. I call this power the Golden Key.

God is omnipotent, and man is His image and likeness, and has dominion over all things. This is the inspired teachings, and it is intended to be taken literally, at its face value. Man means every man, and so the ability to draw on this power is not the prerogative of only the mystic or the saint, as is so often supposed, or even the highly trained practitioner. Whoever you are, wherever you may be, the Golden Key to Internal Physical Fitness and Harmony is in your hand now. You are only the channel through which the divine action takes place. As for the actual method of working, like all fundamental things, it is simplicity itself. All you have to do is this: Stop thinking about the difficulty, whatever it is, and think about Nature and God. It is like coming from the darkness to the light. You can use this power in gaining fitness, in finance, or in anything else conceivable. Whatever it is, just stop thinking about it, and think of God instead. That is all you have to do.

TUNE IN WITH THE INFINITE

Feel that power flowing into every cell of your body. When you are out for a walk, breathe deeply. In the air you are breathing is the breath of God. In the air there is life-sustaining oxygen, but there are other powerful invisible nutrients. That is the reason we called it "the invisible food." You cannot overload on this food. The body will use all you put in —you never gain weight on pure air.

As we purify our bodies and reach INTERNAL PHYSICAL FITNESS, our bodies become receiving instruments for *COSMIC CONSCIOUSNESS*. This means that the higher forces of the universe are flowing through your body. You become one with God and Nature. You are now vibrating on the highest level of consciousness. This tunes you in with the Infinite. You have inexhaustible energy, endurance, strength and vitality. You become one of God's and Nature's perfect children. When you are meditating and when you are out for a hike in the open, use an affirmation like this:

"I am God's perfect child, I am living by God's perfect Laws. Therefore, I have a perfect physical instrument to receive the higher vibrations of the universe." Now, breathe deeply and feel the Divine flow of energy entering your body. That energy is everywhere in the universe. All you have to do is to contact it. You have the *GOLDEN KEYS* for opening your door to INTERNAL PHYSICAL FITNESS, Health and long-lasting Youthfulness.

This is the noble path to enlightment. You are now living a new life because you are working with God and Nature. You have tuned your mind and body with God and Nature. You are now free of fear. You have nothing in the world to fear because you know you are living as God and Nature intended you to live.

IMAGINATION - A POWERFUL FORCE

Remember we are now ruling our life with *MIND-POWER*.

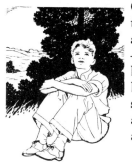
Our minds, not our bodies are ruling. What the mind conceives and believes it can achieve. It is comparatively easy to believe —because it has been proved so—that the body is capable of renewing itself and building new health and youth and strength if given the right food, exercise and care. The mind's part is to accelerate and increase the scope of this progress.

This it can do in many ways. For instance, while you are eating, think of the rejuvenating power which the minerals, vitamins and so on, will release in your glands and organs, and imagine this power at work. When you practise deep breathing, "feel" the life-giving qualities of the air (which, as you know, contains all the elements in vapor form) flooding every cell and tissue; "see" this life filling your whole body as a glowing light. Tell yourself that these things are happening in your body.

Tell yourself you are growing younger and more healthy as often as you can: during the day, and at sleep-time. "See" yourself constantly as you want to be; believe that every day you are growing more like the picture you have made of yourself. Feel young; tell yourself that every muscle is becoming strong and vigorous, and that to move—to be alive, is a joy. Keep this up, day after day.

Perseverance and repetition are two of the chief methods of getting your mind to work for you. MIND-POWER can create miracles for you. And it is worthwhile making the effort to utilize the powers of the subconscious; they are practically limitless, and available to all of us. They can be made use of in many ways—including assistance to the physical exercises in this course.

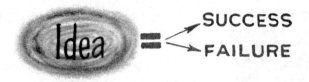

MIND-POWER IN ACTION

The method of doing this is to go through the whole exercise in your mind. See yourself doing the movements; feel your muscles carrying them out. You can do this so intensely that the muscles react almost as if they had actually performed the physical movements. This technique has been used by many people, including a famous long-jump champion. This athlete used to get his trainer to mark out on the ground the distance to be jumped. Then he would lie in a hammock near by, "practicing" his jump mentally. A Hungarian prima donna, whom I knew, sang at the great opera houses of the world without practising a note aloud. She told me that she used to sing her arias over and over again in her mind, "imagining" every note and variation; "hearing" herself singing them. One of the advantages of this method, she said, was that it prevented her voice from becoming fatigued. (Her husband thought it was a good idea too!)

Before I go for a long swim or climb a mountain, in my mind I see myself accomplishing the feat I expect to perform. Once a year I climb Mt. Whitney (the highest mountain in the country except Mt. McKinley, in Alaska.) The night before, I actually visualize myself climbing that mountain and returning without fatigue - but with just a fresh satisfied feeling. Remember, everything is *feel* and *feeling*. We want to *feel* our best at all times!

These are a few examples of what the power of the mind can do for us. But we must not forget that if the mind is to do its best work, it must be properly nourished; just as the body and its organs, including the organ of the mind, the brain, must be given the right food in order to function efficiently. We have discussed the food elements necessary to our physical being, the vitamins and nutrients which the mind needs so it can keep youthful and active. Constructive, positive ideas, "I can" thoughts; plenty of exercise in the way of new concepts and new goals are needed also. The ageing, senile mind, is not the consequence, but one of the causes of the ageing body. Prolonged youth and long life of the body depend chiefly on the condition of the mind or psyche.

BANISH ALL NEGATIVE THOUGHTS

You must never tell yourself you are getting old. You must never tell yourself you are losing your hearing or your eyesight. What you tell yourself actually happens. Many people are old, out of condition, because they kept telling themselves these negative thoughts. Thoughts are living things and you cannot loosely handle thoughts. You are what you think.

Emerson said: "A man is what he thinks all day long!" This is literally true because to think the same type of thought consistently creates an attitude of mind. Eventually this mental attitude affects every cell of the body; it affects the way we move and carry ourselves. So we become what we think; in that sense, we are self-made.

We possess the "Supreme Gift": *THOUGHT!* And depending upon whether we recognize its power and learn to apply it, or neglect it, thought will remake us—or unmake us. So, to learn to control and use the mind and its powers is a pre-requisite of achieving Internal Physical Fitness in its full meaning of developing body, mind and spirit. With the aid of the mind, as science tells us, we can achieve our goal; anything, in fact, upon which we set our hearts.

Begin now to achieve Internal Physical Fitness. Use this tremendous, immediate and ever-available force: Mind-Power. There are no limits to creative power, and the will *of* man.

"TELL OLD AGE TO WAIT!"

In this book, I have tried to bring to your notice the ways, sanctioned by science, past and present, of making yourself Internally Physically Fit. I've tried to show you that, scientifically speaking, I cannot make you fit, young, or happy, or vital. No human being can do that except yourself. All anyone else can do is to point the way. There is no limit to living, according to science. There is a limit only to the will to live . . . the limit you set yourself.

The potentialities of living matter are endless. Protoplasm has been proved potentially immortal. We have seen that the life-span of animals can be increased by additions and shortened by subtractions of "key" elements in the diet. And this finally disposes of the previously unquestioned belief that a life-span was fixed immutably by natural law; that it could be lengthened only by a fluke or shortened only by disease or accident.

As for our own life-span, it certainly is not fixed at three score and ten years, perhaps not even at eight score. But at the moment, we need not look ahead. It is enough, I think, that we can "tell old age to wait." That is the challenge and the victory.

The premature ageing which we now accept as natural has no part in a body with Internal Physical Fitness. The body which is given the right working materials will get on with the job of living, almost indefinitely. The mind which is well-fed will continually function youthfully almost indefinitely. Let me repeat once more that feeding the mind means feeding the brain (its physical organ) with the right vitamins, minerals and nutrients, and also feeding the mind itself with a diet of constructive, positive thoughts which renew and invigorate it. It is just as necessary to sustain the mind in this way as it is to fuel the body with the regular meals.

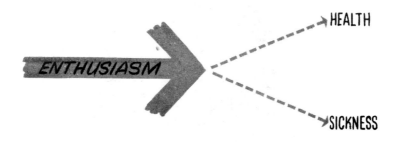

THE MIND—IF YOU DON'T USE IT, YOU LOSE IT

We have to remember, also, that exercise for the mind is just as important as it is for the body. Planned cultivation of the imagination (as described earlier)is one way of exercising the mind; the practice of concentration, which is necessary to the success of any organized mental process, is another. And, above all, the best method of keeping the mind healthy and youthful is to have a purpose of some kind.

To work for a constructive purpose is itself one of the greatest aids to a long healthy life. We all know, or know of, men or women who keep going because they determined to complete some aim or work. Conversely, there are the people who retire to "enjoy life" and die, within a very short time of retirement, because the interest which was the mainspring of their existence is no longer there.

You now have a goal to achieve—you are going to achieve Internal Physical Fitness. Wrap yourself around it; determine to realize your ambition. Now is the time to fall in love with life all over again!

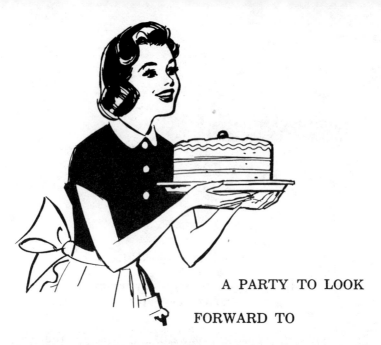

A PARTY TO LOOK
FORWARD TO

The principles about which I have written in this book can be used by anyone. I firmly and fully believe that you and I have within us everything which it takes to enter into the wonderful experience of a fuller, healthier, happier life, that we can begin to do this now, at once, and that we can go on living and enjoying it—well, towards a hundred years or more.

★ ★ ★ ★ ★

Our sincere blessings to you dear friends, who make our lives so worthwhile and fulfilled by reading our teachings on natural living as our Creator laid down for us all to follow . . . Yes—he wants us all to follow the simple path of natural living and this is what we teach in our books and health crusades world-wide. Our prayers reach out to you for the best in health and happiness for you and your loved ones. This is the birthright He gives us all . . . but we must follow the laws He has laid down for us, so we can reap this precious health, physically, mentally and spiritually!

Paul C. Bragg   *Patricia Bragg*

★ ★ ★ ★ ★

"Teach me Thy way, O Lord;
and lead me in a plain path . . ."
Psalms 97:11

94

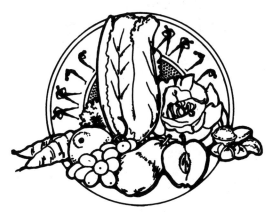

FROM THE AUTHORS

This book was written for YOU. It can be your passport to the Good Life. We Professional Nutritionists join hands in one common objective — a high standard of health for all and many added years to your life. Scientific Nutrition points the way — Nature's Way — the only lasting way to build a body free of degenerative diseases and premature aging. This book teaches you how to work with Nature and not against her. Doctors, dentists, and others who care for the sick, try to repair depleted tissues which too often mend poorly if at all. Many of them praise the spreading of this new scientific message of natural foods and methods for long-lasting health and youthfulness at any age. To speed the spreading of this tremendous message, this book was written.

Statements in this book are recitals of scientific findings, known facts of physiology, biological therapeutics, and reference to ancient writings as they are found. Paul C. Bragg has been practicing the natural methods of living for over 70 years, with highly beneficial results, knowing they are safe and of great value to others, and his daughter Patricia Bragg works with him to carry on the Health Crusade. They make no claims as to what the methods cited in this book will do for one in any given situation, and assume no obligation because of opinions expressed.

No cure for disease is offered in this book. No foods or diets are offered for the treatment or cure of any specific ailment. Nor is it intended as, or to be used as, literature for any food product. Paul C. Bragg and Patricia Bragg express their opinions solely as Public Health Educators, Professional Nutritionists and Teachers.

Certain persons considered experts may disagree with one or more statements in this book, as the same relate to various nutritional recommendations. However, any such statements are considered, nevertheless, to be factual, as based upon long-time experience of Paul C. Bragg and Patricia Bragg in the field of human health.

SEND FOR IMPORTANT
FREE HEALTH BULLETINS

Patricia Bragg, from time to time sends News Bulletins on latest Health and Nutrition Discoveries. These are sent *free of charge!*

The Health Builder, the magazine devoted to Nutrition and Physical Fitness, is also sent *free* to those who are interested in gaining and maintaining superb health!

If you wish to receive these *free bulletins* and The Health Builder— please send your name and also names of any friends and relatives you wish.

HEALTH SCIENCE Box 7, Santa Barbara, California 93102 U.S.A.

Name

Address

City   State   Zip Code

Name

Address

City   State   Zip Code

Name

Address

City   State   Zip Code

Name

Address

City   State   Zip Code